FUNDAMENTALS OF FLUOROSCOPY

FUNDAMENTALS OF Fluoroscopy

Jeffrey D. Houston, M.D.

Department of Radiology

University of New Mexico Health Sciences Center

Albuquerque, New Mexico

Michael Davis, M.D.

Professor Emeritus of Radiology and Past Chief of

Gastrointestinal and Genitourinary Radiology

Department of Radiology

University of New Mexico Health Sciences Center

Albuquerque, New Mexico

W.B. SAUNDERS COMPANY

A Harcourt Health Sciences Company

Philadelphia London New York St. Louis Sydney Toronto

W.B. Saunders Company
A Harcourt Health Sciences Company
The Curtis Center
Independence Square West
Philadelphia, Pennsylvania 19106

Library of Congress Cataloging-in-Publication Data

Houston, Jeffrey D.
Fundamentals of fluoroscopy / Jeffrey D. Houston, Michael Davis.—1st ed.
p. ; cm.
ISBN 0-7216-9407-1
1. Diagnosis, Fluoroscopic—Handbooks, manuals, etc. I. Davis, Michael, 1940–
II. Title.
[DNLM: 1. Fluoroscopy—Handbooks. WN 39 H843f2001]
RC78.7.F5 H68 2001
616.07'572—dc21

2001032257

FUNDAMENTALS OF FLUOROSCOPY ISBN 0-7216-9407-1

Printed in the United States of America

Last digit is the print number: 9 8 7 6 5 4 3 2 1

To my parents
and the residents
who inspired this book
JDH

To Gae
MD

Contributors

Michael Davis, M.D.
Professor Emeritus and Past Chief of Gastrointestinal and Genitourinary Radiology
Department of Radiology
University of New Mexico Health Sciences Center
Albuquerque, New Mexico

Jeffrey D. Houston, M.D.
Department of Radiology
University of New Mexico Health Sciences Center
Albuquerque, New Mexico

Charles A. Kelsey, Ph.D.
Professor and Chief of Biomedical Physics
Department of Radiology
University of New Mexico Health Sciences Center
Albuquerque, New Mexico

Thomas P. Martin, M.D.
Associate Professor and Chief of Musculoskeletal Radiology
Department of Radiology
University of New Mexico Health Sciences Center
Albuquerque, New Mexico

Brock G. McDaniel, M.D.
Department of Radiology
University of New Mexico Health Sciences Center
Albuquerque, New Mexico

Frederick W. Rupp, M.D.
Associate Professor
Department of Radiology
University of New Mexico Health Sciences Center
Albuquerque, New Mexico

Philip W. Wiest, M.D.
Associate Professor and Chief of Gastrointestinal and Genitourinary Radiology
Department of Radiology
University of New Mexico Health Sciences Center
Albuquerque, New Mexico

Preface

Over the past three years, this manual has grown from a twelve-page tutorial on four basic fluoroscopic exams for first-year radiology residents to an inclusive procedural handbook of noninterventional fluoroscopy. We discovered that we had developed something useful when we could no longer maintain a supply of spare copies of the book. After they were printed, copies were quickly requested by technologists, medical students, residents, and attending radiologists.

Our goals are twofold: to provide a framework for the beginning radiology resident to develop a systematic approach for performing fluoroscopic exams and to provide a quick reference for the experienced radiologist when performing uncommon procedures.

Most of the fluoroscopic exams that a radiologist will encounter are listed. We strive to outline the indications for performing the exam, the necessary equipment and technical factors, and the basic sequence of films that should be obtained. Techniques for both conventional and digital fluoroscopy are provided. Obviously, exams demonstrating abnormal findings often require obtaining various additional images.

We have designed the book to be practical, compact, and concise. Thus, we have intentionally omitted discussions of pathology that can be seen when performing the exams. We have consequently limited our handbook to providing examples of how routine exams should be performed.

The following are our protocols for performing fluoroscopic exams. These protocols have been used successfully for many years at the University of New Mexico. It has been said that if two radiologists are consulted on a single case, three opinions will be rendered. Likewise, there are many individual preferences on how these exams should be performed. Our protocols are certainly not the only ways of performing the exams and should be used as a framework, with exams modified as needed for individual circumstances.

Jeffrey D. Houston
Michael Davis

Acknowledgments

A compilation of this size has invariably received input from many individuals. Foremost, we thank the resident radiologists at the University of New Mexico Health Sciences Center, who inspired us to write this handbook. Their helpful suggestions have been integral in creating a concise and understandable framework for describing the procedures.

We thank Susan L. Williamson, M.D., for her assistance in reviewing the pediatric radiology exams. Charles A. Kelsey, Ph.D., deserves credit for providing the radiation doses listed throughout the book. Many of the images could not have been obtained without the contributions of our colleagues and the assistance of the departmental technologists, particularly Paul Gonzales, R.T.

We especially thank Charlotte Hendrix and Joseph Tafoya for their valuable assistance in editing and assembling the manuscript and processing the images. Charlotte has gone far beyond the call of duty in managing the production of this book, and without her help, the book probably would never have been completed. Finally, we commend Lisette Bralow and her staff at W.B. Saunders Company and Peggy Gordon and her staff at P.M. Gordon Associates for their expertise, professionalism, and valuable contributions to this project.

Contents

Introduction

How to Use This Handbook

The following examination protocols are intended for adult patients unless otherwise specified. Each fluoroscopic examination is introduced by listing common indications and contraindications, suggested patient preparation, required and optional supplies, recommended scout film, sample dictation, estimated radiation dose, and representative images of pertinent radiographic anatomy. Tables of fluoroscopic supplies, including generic and trade names (and manufacturers), can be found in the appendices.

The protocols for the following exams are listed step by step in table format. We have found that this format is the most straightforward method of communicating all the factors that must be considered for successfully performing each step of the exam. The left column contains representative images and the suggested film sizes and layouts. The instructions for each step are listed in the center column. The right column contains positioning information as it pertains to the fluoroscope tabletop and the patient, as well as additional suggested technical factors.

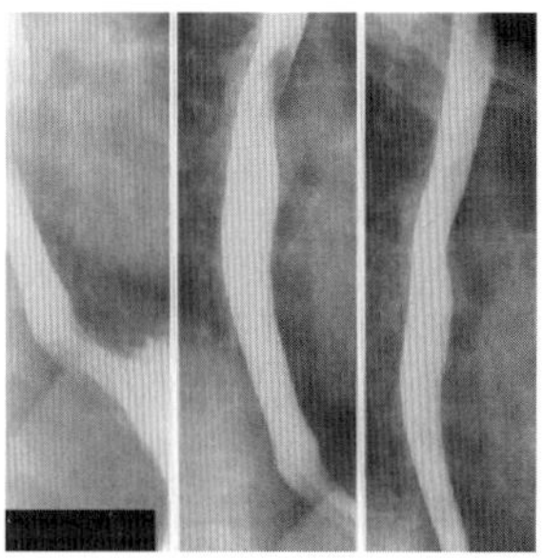

14 × 14
3 on 1
or
spot film
±mag

1 *Image Entire Esophagus*

Have the patient continuously drink the regular barium to fill and distend the esophagus, while images are obtained of:

1. The proximal esophagus
2. The midesophagus
3. The distal esophagus, including an open lower esophageal sphincter (magnified if possible)

TABLETOP
Head Down
−20°

110 kVp

PATIENT
RAO/LPO

FIGURE 1. *Sample of formatting used to describe the steps for performing each exam.*

Suggested film sizes for fluoroscopic procedures mainly include 10 × 12 inch and 14 × 14 inch cassettes, although these sizes may need to be adapted for individual fluoroscopes. Some modern fluoroscopes produce only digital spot films, for which the magnification factors can be manipulated to control the size of the field of view. Common film layouts are 3 on 1 (vertical), 2 on 1 (vertical and horizontal), and 1 on 1.

Technical factor abbreviations that appear in the right column include

- kVp (for increased conspicuity, suggested kVp is listed only at the beginning of the procedure and when a change in technique or imaging modality occurs)
- rapid seq (rapid sequence imaging and suggested frame rates are listed in each step when recommended)
- pulsed fluoro (digital pulsed fluoroscopy and suggested frame rates are recommended for some entire exams and are listed only at the beginning of the procedure)

Symbols that will be encountered include

[●][▶] —indicates that the step should be recorded using a videocassette recorder

℞—indicates drug administration. Abbreviations for routes of administration are

IV (intravenous)
sc (subcutaneous)
IM (intramuscular)

Variations of some routine examinations for specific conditions are designated by the ✪ symbol and follow the steps for the accompanying routine exam.

The fluoroscopic dose rate used in the listed dose estimates is 3000 mrad/min. If the dose rate of your machines differs appreciably from this value, a corresponding modification to the doses given for the various examinations should be made.

Radiation doses are reported as effective doses. The effective dose takes into account not only the amount of radiation but also the organs that are irradiated. More information regarding the effective dose concept can be found in the National Council on Radiation Protection and Measurements Report Number 112, "Use of Personal Monitors to Estimate Effective Dose Equivalent and Effective Dose to Workers for External Exposure to Low LET Radiation, December 1995" (National Council on Radiation Protection and Measurements, 7910 Woodmont Ave., Bethesda, MD, 20814-3095).

These examinations should be performed only by trained radiologists and radiology technologists. A brief medical history should be obtained from all patients, including specific questions regarding the possibility of pregnancy and allergies to radiologic contrast media or other medications. A common premedication algorithm can be found in the appendices for patients with a history of a mild contrast reaction. Every fluoroscopy suite should have immediate accessibility to emergency medical supplies, including but not limited to medications for treating allergic reactions to contrast media.

Fluoroscopy Tabletop Positions

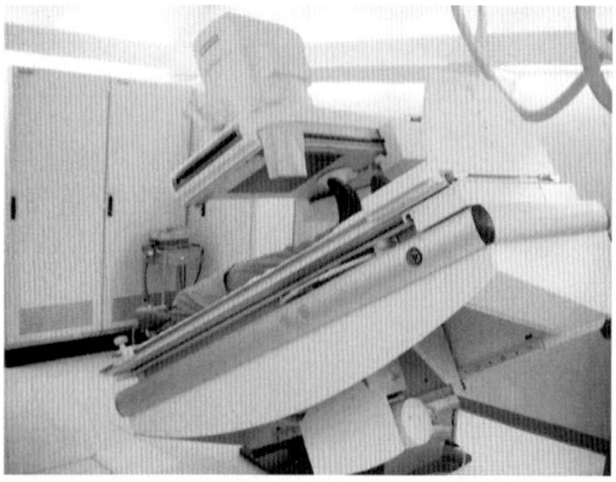

Head Down *(−45°)*

The fluoroscopy tabletop is declined, with the patient supported by shoulder rests that are secured to the tabletop.

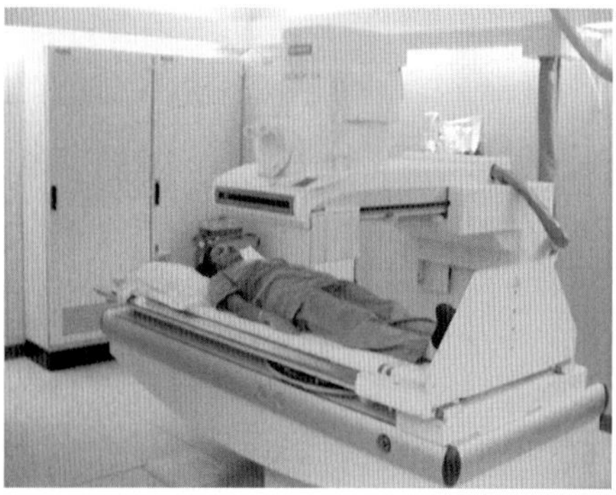

Horizontal *(0°)*

The fluoroscopy tabletop is placed in the horizontal position.

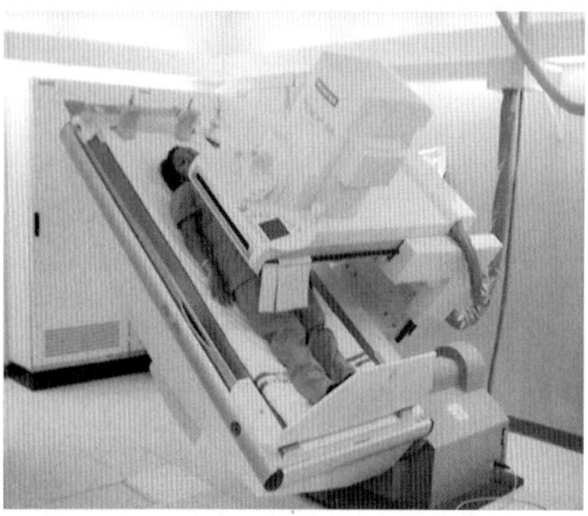

Head Up *(45°)*

The fluoroscopy tabletop is elevated, with the patient supported by a footboard that is secured to the tabletop.

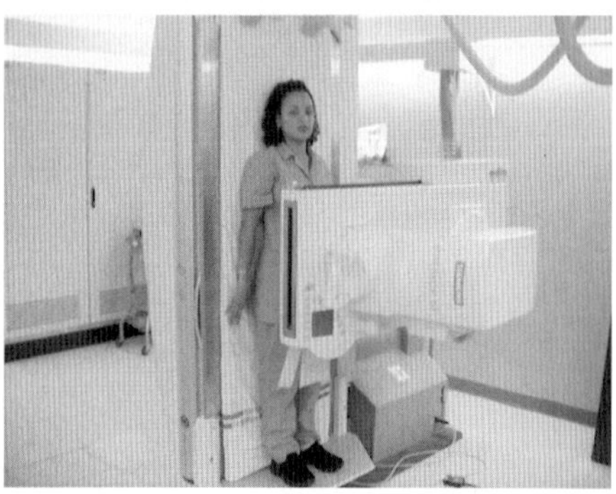

Vertical *(90°)*

The fluoroscopy tabletop is elevated to the vertical position, with the patient standing or sitting on a footboard that is secured to the tabletop.

Patient Positions

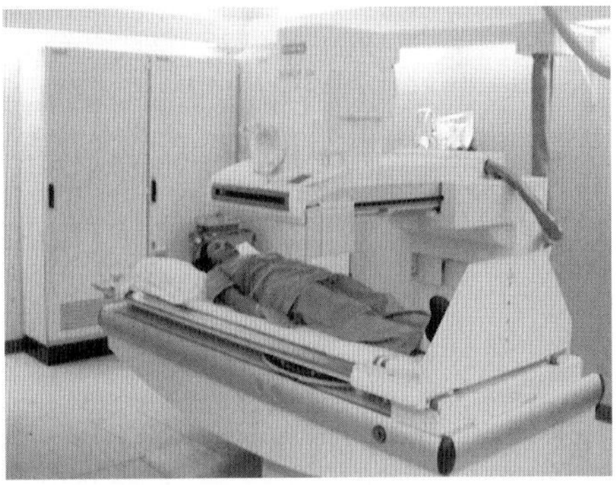

AP *(Anteroposterior)*

The patient is placed supine on the fluoroscopy tabletop.

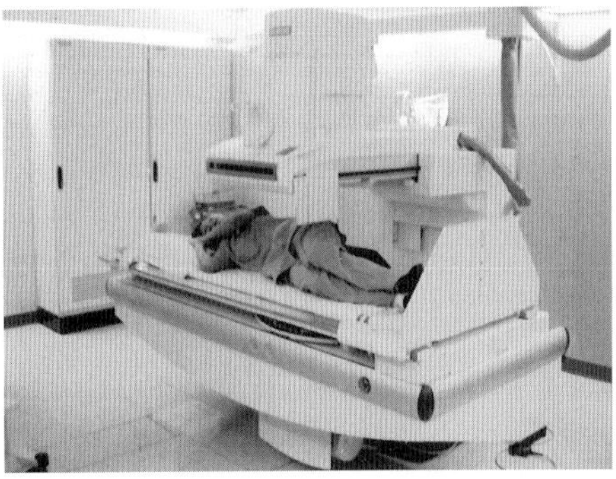

RPO *(Right Posterior Oblique)*

The patient is placed supine on the fluoroscopy tabletop and rotated 45° to the right.

A triangular foam wedge may be placed under the patient's back.

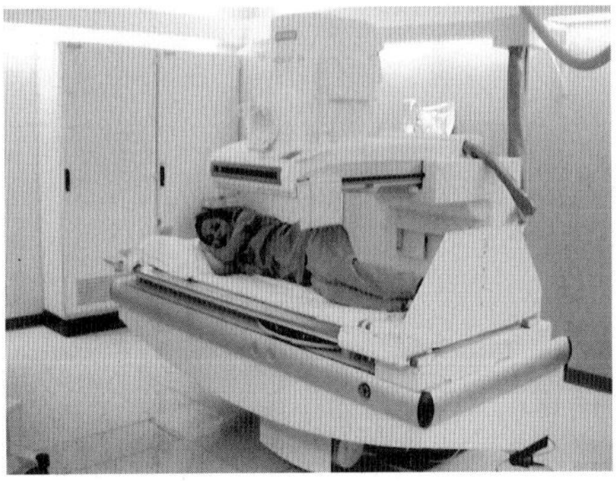

Rt Lat *(Right Lateral)*

The patient is placed perpendicular to the fluoroscopy tabletop with the right side down.

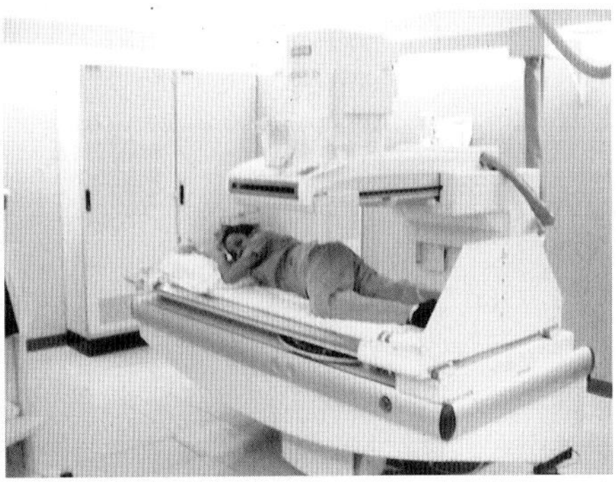

RAO *(Right Anterior Oblique)*

The patient is placed prone on the fluoroscopy tabletop and rotated 45° to the right.

A triangular foam wedge may be placed under the patient's abdomen.

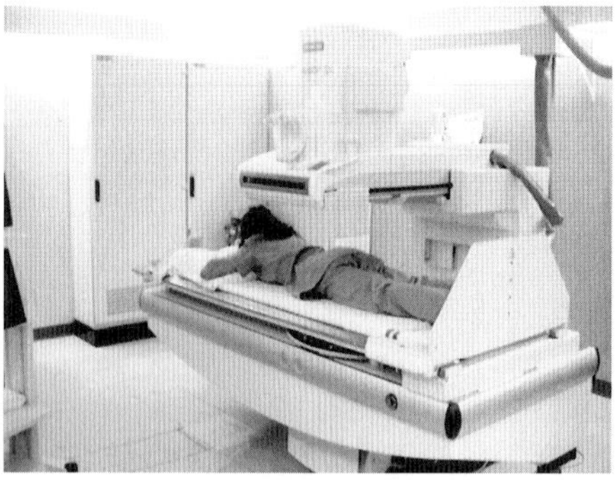

PA *(Posteroanterior)*

The patient is placed prone on the fluoroscopy tabletop.

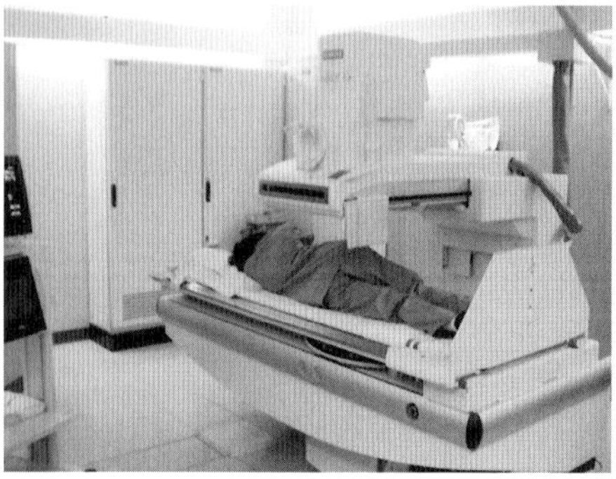

LAO *(Left Anterior Oblique)*

The patient is placed prone on the fluoroscopy tabletop and rotated 45° to the left.

A triangular foam wedge may be placed under the patient's abdomen.

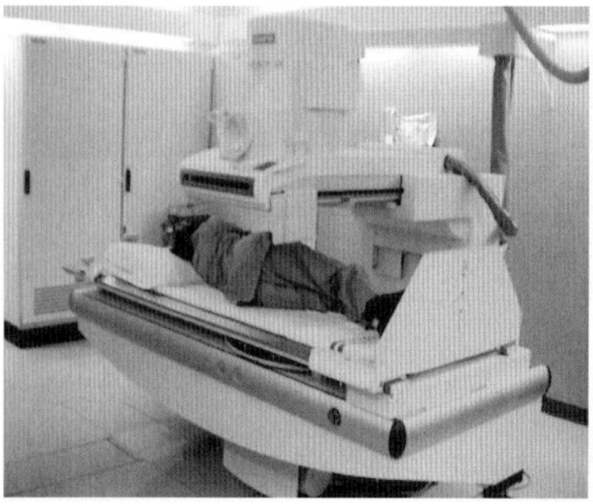

Lt Lat *(Left Lateral)*

The patient is placed perpendicular to the fluoroscopy tabletop with the left side down.

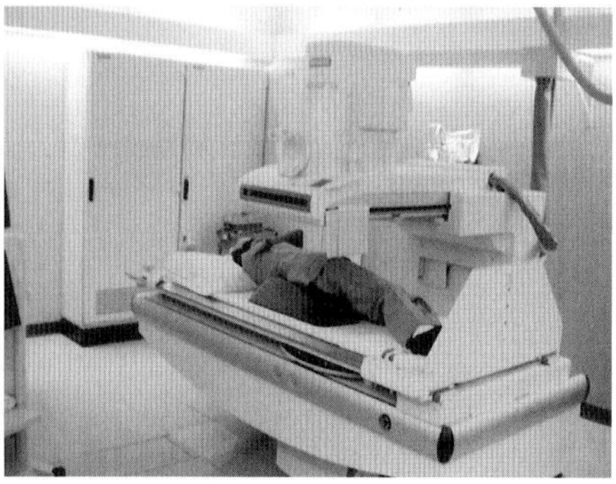

LPO *(Left Posterior Oblique)*

The patient is placed supine on the fluoroscopy tabletop and rotated 45° to the left.

A triangular foam wedge may be placed under the patient's back.

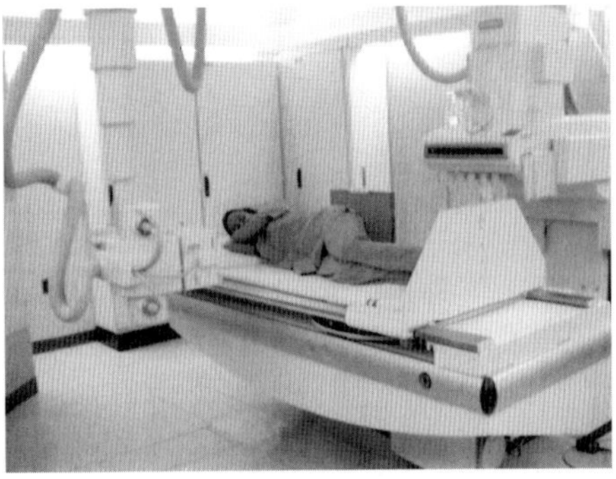

RLD *(Right Lateral Decubitus)*

The patient is placed perpendicular to the fluoroscopy tabletop with the right side down. X-rays are directed parallel to the tabletop from a ceiling-mounted tube.

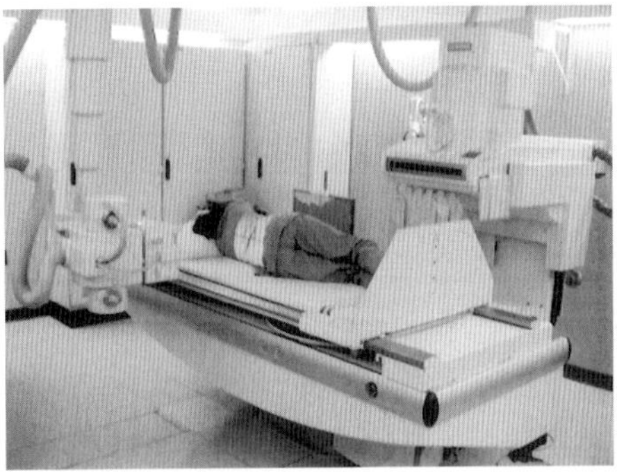

LLD *(Left Lateral Decubitus)*

The patient is placed perpendicular to the fluoroscopy tabletop with the left side down. X-rays are directed parallel to the tabletop from a ceiling-mounted tube.

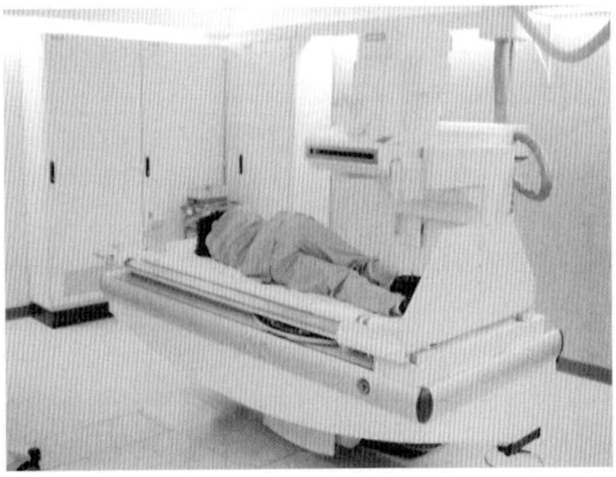

Sims

The patient is placed in the LAO position with the right knee and hip flexed.

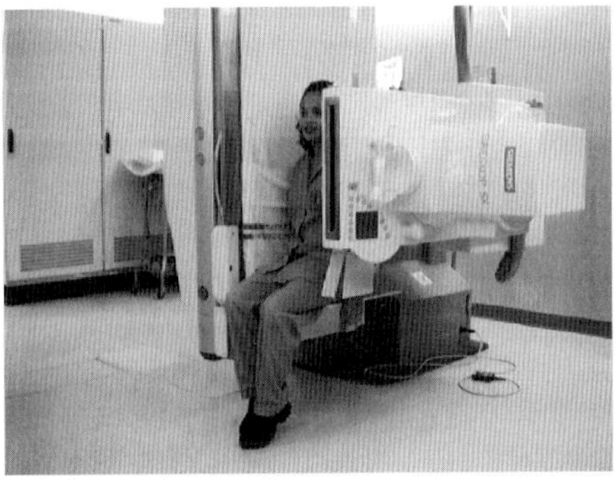

Sitting

With the tabletop positioned vertically, the patient sits on the fluoroscopy footboard.

Pregnancy and Radiation

Charles A. Kelsey, Ph.D.

If a patient is pregnant, the first thought should be whether an alternative examination that does not require ionizing radiation, such as endoscopy, magnetic resonance imaging, or ultrasound, is available. As a matter of policy at many institutions, only patients undergoing radiographic examinations that could produce doses greater than 2 mGy (200 mrad) to the fetus are considered to be at any risk from radiation. This value was chosen because it is 40% less than the allowed fetal dose recommended by NCRP Report 116, "Limitation of Exposure to Ionizing Radiation" (SCRP II 6) for pregnant workers. This section will discuss the expected radiation dose and potential hazard to the fetus from those examinations that may produce fetal radiation doses greater than 2 mGy.

The possible risks will be presented in two parts: (1) the radiation dose compared to years of living in a high background radiation location and (2) chances of the child developing a fatal cancer.

Background Radiation

The background radiation level of a representative Western city at an elevation of 5000 feet is approximately 4 mGy (400 mrad) per year or roughly 80 μGy/week (8 mrad). Half of this amount is from radon; the other half is divided among cosmic, terrestrial, and internal sources. The fetus does not receive the radon dose.

For example, an examination resulting in a fetal dose of 4 mGy would be compared to the dose received by a person living for 12 months in Denver, Colorado. The following examples use this dose equivalent for calculation purposes.

Loss of Life Expectancy

In comparing the risk from radiation to other risks, the concept of loss of life expectancy (LLE) is used. Participating in a risky activity will reduce a person's life expectancy. The LLE is a way of estimating the average risk of an activity. Life expectancy in the United States depends on many factors but is about 70 years. As an example of the concept of LLE, consider skydiving. In 1991 there were 4.8 million skydiving jumps. Seventy-four deaths occurred during that year. If all the jumpers who died were age 30, and on the average each would have lived to age 70, each jumper killed is assumed to have lost 40 years of life expectancy or a total of 26 million hours of life expectancy. This LLE can be averaged over the 4.8 million jumps to yield an LLE of 5.4 hours LLE per jump.

The second way to express risk in terms of LLE is based on the risk of excess weight. Being 15% overweight results in an expected loss of life of 770 days. Cohen and Lee* equate an exposure of 10 mGy to an LLE of 1.5 days. This is based on the linear nonthreshold (LNT) model of radiation response. There is considerable discussion of the validity of this model, but we use it because it is convenient, easy to use, and probably conservative (overestimates the risk).

Chances of Developing Cancer

The third way to describe the risk to the fetus from an examination is to estimate how much the chance of developing a fatal cancer increases because of the examination. Calculations of the increased chance that a child will develop a fatal cancer are based on extrapolations of data obtained at high radiation doses and compared to the much lower doses in radiographic examinations.

In estimates of the increased chance of the fetus developing a fatal cancer, it can be assumed that the fetus is twice as sensitive to radiation damage as an adult. The natural incidence of fatal cancer or leukemia reveals that of 10,000 babies born in the Unites States, 2000 will develop a fatal cancer in their lifetime. This is a fatal cancer incidence rate of 20%. If 10,000 pregnant mothers get an examination, estimates can be made as to how many additional cancer

* Cohen BL, Lee IS. A catalog of risks. *Health Phys* 1979; 36:707–722.

deaths will be expected in their offspring due to the radiation from the examination. The cancer risk used in preparing these estimates is based on an assumption of an additional 10 cancer deaths per 10,000 babies exposed in utero to 10 mGy (1000 mrad).

Diagnostic Procedures

Interventional fluoroscopic or computed tomography (CT) procedures are not included in this manual but can certainly result in significant radiation doses. Only noninterventional diagnostic procedures resulting in fetal doses greater than 2 mGy are covered. Routine diagnostic examinations to non-pregnant patients involve negligible risk or hazard. Diagnostic procedures that may produce fetal doses greater than 2 mGy include:

- Abdominal and pelvic radiography
- Intravenous urography
- Barium enema
- Pelvic CT
- Lumbosacral spine radiography
- Interventional procedures

All radiology facilities should be prepared to provide estimates of radiation doses (expressed as the effective dose) and the risks from any examination to any patient who requests this information. It is usually not necessary to provide dose estimates for nonpregnant patients undergoing routine diagnostic examinations.

Shielding of pregnant patients is almost never necessary. It is contraindicated if the uterus is in the field to be examined because the shielding will obscure the area of interest. If the uterus is not in the x-ray field, the only radiation reaching the fetus is internal scattered radiation. External shielding of the patient's skin surface will not attenuate the internal scattered radiation. Providing an external lead shield will make the patient feel better and will demonstrate the institution's concern for her protection. In many institutions this is sufficient justification for providing such shields.

Radiation risks from representative examinations described in this book are discussed below.

Abdominal and Pelvic Radiographs

The risks from these abdominal and pelvic radiographs are additive. If a patient is receiving more than one of these examinations, the risk from all the examinations must be added together to obtain the total risk. An abdominal, kidney-ureters-bladder (KUB), or pelvic radiographic examination gives a fetal dose of about 2 mGy. To put this dose in perspective:

1. The fetus will receive from this examination the same amount of radiation we receive through natural background radiation over a period of 6 months.
2. The fetus may lose 14 hours of life expectancy as a result of this examination.
3. The natural incidence of cancer is 2000 out of every 10,000 babies born. If 10,000 pregnant mothers get this examination, we expect 2 extra cancers in their children for a total of 2002 cancers.

Barium Enema

The risks from these examinations are additive. If a patient is receiving more than one of these examinations, the risk from all the examinations must be added together to obtain the total risk. The barium enema exam gives a fetal dose of about 9 mGy (900 mrad).

1. The fetus will receive from this examination the same amount of radiation we receive through natural background radiation over a period of 2.25 years.
2. The fetus may lose 64 hours of life expectancy as a result of this examination.
3. The natural incidence of cancer deaths is 2000 out of every 10,000 babies born. If 10,000 pregnant mothers get this examination, we expect 10 extra cancer deaths in their children for a total of 2010 cancer deaths.

Intravenous Urography

The risks from these examinations are additive. If a patient is receiving more than one of these examinations, the risk from all the examinations must be added together to obtain the total risk. An intravenous pyelography (IVP) exam gives a fetal dose of 6 mGy (600 mrad).

1. The fetus will receive from this examination the same amount of radiation we receive through natural background radiation over a period of 1.5 years.
2. The fetus may lose 43 hours of life expectancy as a result of this examination.

3. The natural incidence of cancer deaths is 2000 out of every 10,000 babies born. If 10,000 pregnant mothers get this examination, we expect 6 additional cancer deaths in their children for a total of 2006 cancer deaths.

Conclusion

As discussed above, the risks associated with many routine radiologic examinations in pregnancy are relatively nominal, but can be significantly increased with repeat examinations, additional radiographic exposures, or prolonged fluoroscopy times. However, because of the risks to the fetus, the decision to perform any examination requiring ionizing radiation should be carefully weighed with respect to its medical necessity, urgency, and lack of alternative imaging modalities, such as ultrasound, magnetic resonance imaging, or endoscopy.

At our institution, all women of childbearing age are asked if they could possibly be pregnant before undergoing radiologic examination. If the patient is determined to be pregnant, the decision to proceed with the examination can be reassessed. If it is determined that performing the examination is medically necessary despite the risks and no nonradiation alternative is available, informed and written consent is obtained from the patient, if possible. Considering terminating the pregnancy is not recommended for fetal doses less than 1000 mGy (10 rad), which are rarely if ever needed during fluoroscopy. Performing a barium enema or IVP on a woman later discovered to be pregnant is never reason to terminate a pregnancy.

Pharmaceuticals

The following are brief synopses of the most common drugs used for fluoroscopic procedures. See the package inserts for more complete details.

Glucagon

H_2N-His-Ser-Gln-Gly-Thr-Phe-Thr-Ser-Asp-Tyr-Ser-Lys-Tyr-Leu-Asp-Ser-Arg-Arg-Ala-Gln-Asp-Phe-Val-Gln-Trp-Leu-Met-Asn-Thr-COOH

description: A single-chain polypeptide normally produced by the α-cells of the pancreas. Glucagon mobilizes hepatic glycogen and converts it to glucose, and is most commonly used to treat hypoglycemia in diabetics. Glucagon relaxes the smooth muscle of the stomach, duodenum, small bowel, and colon. This relaxation is the basis of its usage in gastrointestinal radiologic procedures to reduce spasm and motion artifact and to cause temporary paralysis of the gut.

dosage: In adults, 0.1 to 1.0 mg is administered intravenously (onset within 1 minute) or intramuscularly (onset within 10 minutes). Reconstituted glucagon should be used immediately after preparation. Depending on the route of administration, the duration of action is up to 20 minutes.

manufacturer: Glucagon (Lilly) lyophilized powder with diluent.

adverse reactions: Nausea, vomiting, abdominal pain, hypersensitivity reactions.

drug interactions: Glucagon has an effect opposite to that of insulin.

contraindications: Pheochromocytoma, insulinoma, known hypersensitivity to glucagon. Hypertensive crisis can result in pheochromocytoma owing to release of catecholamines by the tumor. Intravenous phentolamine (5–10 mg) can be used to attempt to control blood pressure. Rebound hypoglycemia can occur in patients with insulinomas and can be treated with oral or intravenous glucose.

Lidocaine Hydrochloride

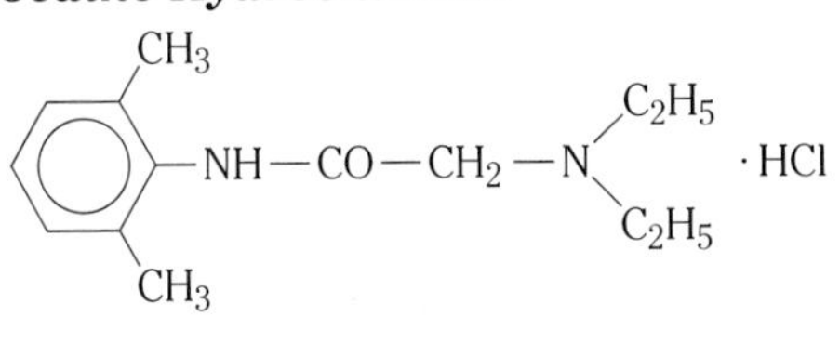

description: A parenterally injected local anesthetic that stabilizes the neuronal membrane by inhibiting ionic fluxes required for neural impulses. Lidocaine is available in various concentrations, with and without epinephrine.

dosage: To avoid intravascular injection, aspiration should always be performed before injection to check for blood return. For percutaneous infiltration, a 1% solution is recommended. When used without epinephrine in healthy adults, the maximum dose should not exceed 4.5 mg/kg and a total dose of 300 mg. With epinephrine, the maximum dose should not exceed 7 mg/kg and a total dose of 500 mg.

manufacturer: Various ampules/vials with and without epinephrine and preservatives

Xylocaine (AstraZeneca)
Lidocaine HCl injection (Baxter, Elkins-Sinn)

adverse reactions: Generally result from high plasma levels and include CNS effects, bradycardia, hypotension, cardiovascular collapse, allergic reaction to anesthetic or preservative.

drug interactions: Most drug interactions are secondary to solutions containing epinephrine.

contraindications: Intravascular injection, known hypersensitivity to amide local anesthetics.

Metoclopramide Hydrochloride

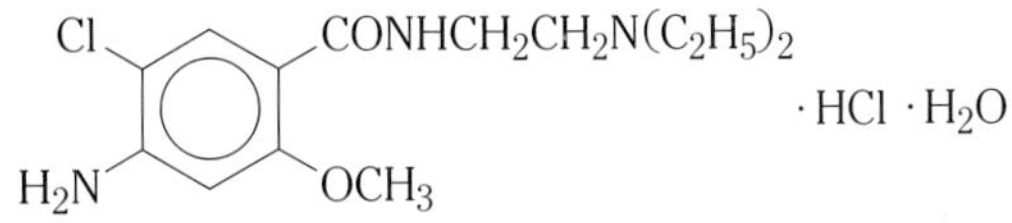

description: A dopamine receptor antagonist that increases lower esophageal sphincter pressure, increases the rate of gastric emptying, and stimulates motility of the upper gastrointestinal tract. Metoclopramide is commonly used in the treatment of diabetic gastroparesis and has been used in treating gastroesophageal reflux.

dosage: Although effectively absorbed orally, the onset of action (30–60 minutes) by this route makes it suboptimal for radiologic use. Therefore, it is routinely administered intramuscularly or intravenously (over 30–60 seconds, as rapid administration can be associated with transient anxiety and restlessness followed by drowsiness):

adults—10 mg (2 mL)
children 6–14 years—2.5 to 5 mg (0.5 to1 mL)
children under 6 years—0.1 mg/kg

Onset of action is 1–3 minutes when administered intravenously and 10–15 minutes following intramuscular administration.

manufacturers:
Reglan Injectable (Robins)
Metoclopramide Injection (Baxter)

adverse reactions: Adverse reactions include drowsiness, lassitude, anxiety, and changes in blood pressure. Hypertensive crisis can result in patients with pheochromocytoma.

drug interactions: Use should be avoided in patients who have received monoamine oxidase inhibitors or tricyclic antidepressants within the previous 2 weeks.

contraindications: Known hypersensitivity to metoclopramide, pheochromocytoma, mechanical obstruction, perforation, and gastrointestinal hemorrhage. It is not recommended in patients with extrapyramidal symptoms or epilepsy. Hypertensive crisis can result in patients with pheochromocytoma owing to release of catecholamines by the tumor. Intravenous phentolamine (5–10 mg) can be used to attempt to control blood pressure.

Sincalide

SO_3H
|
Asp–Tyr–Met–Gly–Trp–Met–Asp–Phe–NH_2

description: The C-terminal octapeptide of cholecystokinin. Sincalide causes prompt gallbladder contraction, similar to the physiologic response to endogenous cholecystokinin. It has maximal effect 5 to 15 minutes after intravenous administration.

dosage: In adults, 0.02 μg/kg is administered intravenously over 30–60 seconds. Reconstituted sincalide should be used within 24 hours of preparation. If satisfactory gallbladder contraction does not occur in 15 minutes, a second dose of 0.04 μg/kg can be administered.

manufacturer: Kinevac (Bracco) lyophilized powder.

adverse reactions: Nausea, abdominal pain.

drug interactions: No known interactions.

contraindications: Bowel obstruction, known hypersensitivity to sincalide, pregnancy near term.

PART I

Pharyngeal and Esophageal Examinations

Michael Davis, M.D.
Jeffrey D. Houston, M.D.

Videofluoroscopic Swallowing Exam

INDICATIONS

- Dysphagia (difficulty swallowing)
- Odynophagia (painful swallowing)
- Globus (sensation of a lump in the throat)
- Suspected aspiration
- Postoperative assessment of laryngectomy
- Penetrating trauma

CONTRAINDICATIONS

- If pharyngeal perforation is suspected, water-soluble contrast is used by convention.
- If aspiration or a fistula to the airway is suspected, ionic water-soluble contrast is avoided.

PATIENT PREPARATION

- None

SUPPLIES

- 4–6 oz dense barium (200–250% w/v)
- Barium cup
- Suction should be available if the patient is unable to clear the airway of aspirated contents.

SCOUT FILM

- Not obtained routinely

SAMPLE DICTATION

Videofluoroscopic swallowing evaluation was performed using dense barium. Oral transit was normal. No significant pooling was evident in the valleculae or pyriform sinuses. There was no evidence of nasopharyngeal reflux, laryngeal penetration, or frank tracheal aspiration. No cricopharyngeal abnormalities were noted. The pharynx and cervical spine have a normal appearance. ■

RADIATION

- Fluoro: 325 mrad/min

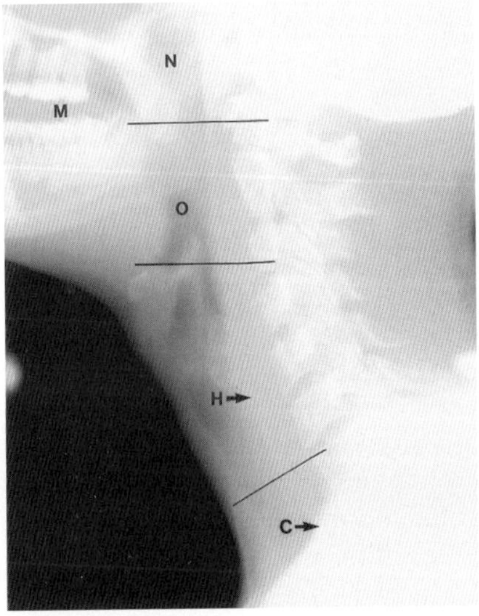

M—mouth (oral cavity) (from lips to uvula)

N—nasopharynx (posterior to soft palate, extending from skull base through uvula)

O—oropharynx (from tip of uvula to hyoid bone)

H—hypopharynx (from hyoid bone to pharyngoesophageal junction)

C—cervical esophagus (from pharyngoesophageal junction to thoracic inlet)

FIGURE 1. *Anatomic divisions of the pharynx.*

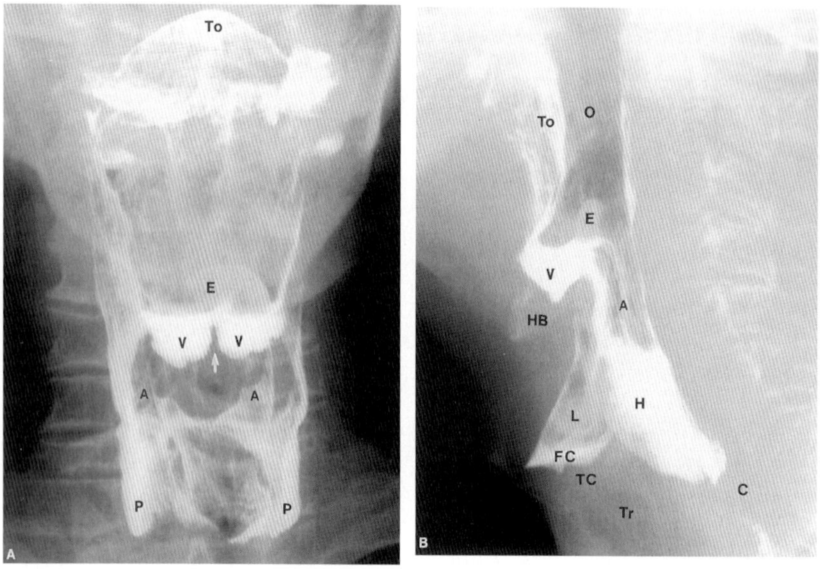

O—oropharynx
To—base of tongue
E—epiglottis
V—valleculae
A—aryepiglottic folds
P—pyriform recesses
HB—hyoid bone
H—hypopharynx
L—larynx
FC—false cords
TC—true cords
Tr—trachea
C—cricopharyngeus muscle
arrow—median glossoepiglottic fold

FIGURE 2. *Pharyngeal anatomy. Abnormal AP (A) and lateral (B) swallowing exams allow visualization of anatomy that is usually not completely visualized. Vallecular pooling, mild hyopharyngeal dilatation, laryngeal penetration, and cricopharyngeal hypertrophy are all present.*

EXAM

1 *Prepare Video Recorder*

Record the entire exam on videotape (if available) or use rapid sequence spot filming at the highest frame rate possible (minimum four frames/sec). To coordinate imaging with the swallow, the radiologist should give the following count: "1 . . . 2 . . . 3 . . . swallow." This allows some video recorders to come up to speed, as the technologist starts recording on "1." As each swallow occurs, do not move the fluoroscope.

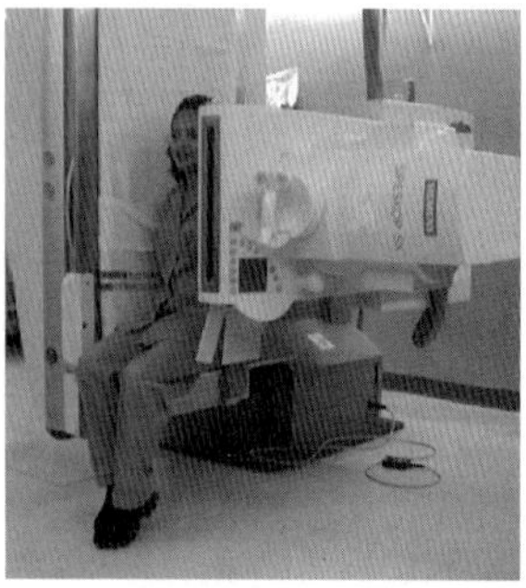

2 *Position Patient*

The patient may either stand or sit on the footboard in the right lateral position, with the neck slightly extended. Immobile patients can be placed in a fluoroscopy chair, which can be rolled into position between the tabletop and tower or secured to the footboard. If necessary, this exam can be performed with the patient in a gurney, using a C-arm fluoroscope.

TABLETOP
Vertical

PATIENT
Rt Lat

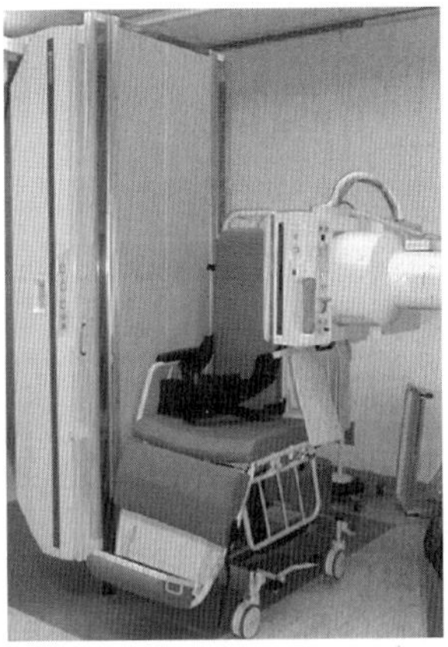

2 *Position Patient* *(continued)*

Collimate as needed to focus on the soft tissues and remove the air gap that can degenerate the image.

Place the cup of barium in the patient's right hand. Ask the patient to fill the mouth with barium but to refrain from swallowing until instructed to do so.

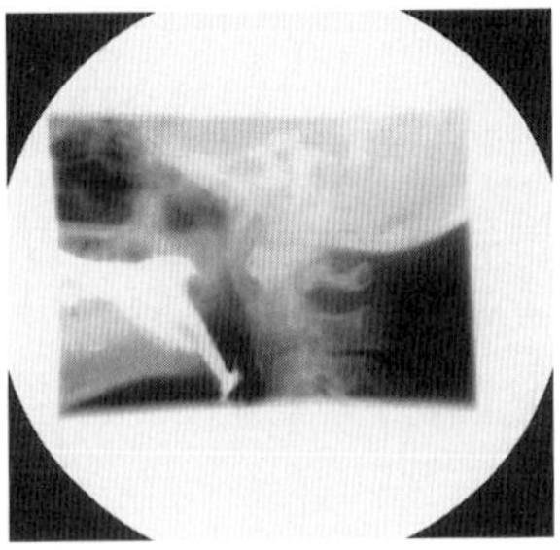

3 *Image Lateral Oral Cavity and Nasopharynx*

On the first swallow, imaging should focus on the mouth and nasopharynx.

TABLETOP

Vertical

110 kVp

PATIENT

Rt Lat

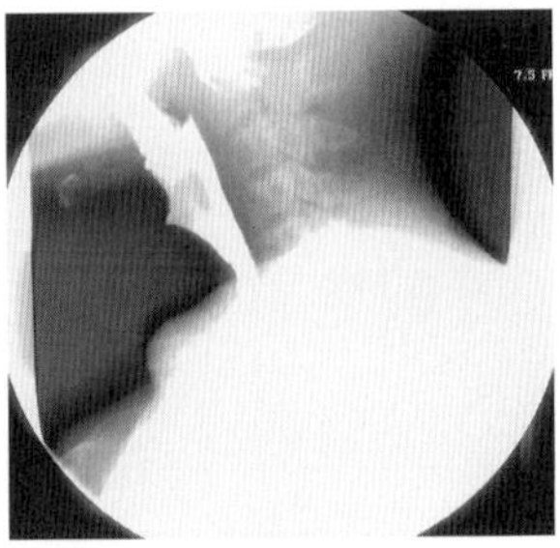

4 *Image Lateral Oropharynx*

The second swallow should focus on the oropharynx, which extends from the soft palate inferiorly to the hyoid bone.

TABLETOP

Vertical

PATIENT

Rt Lat

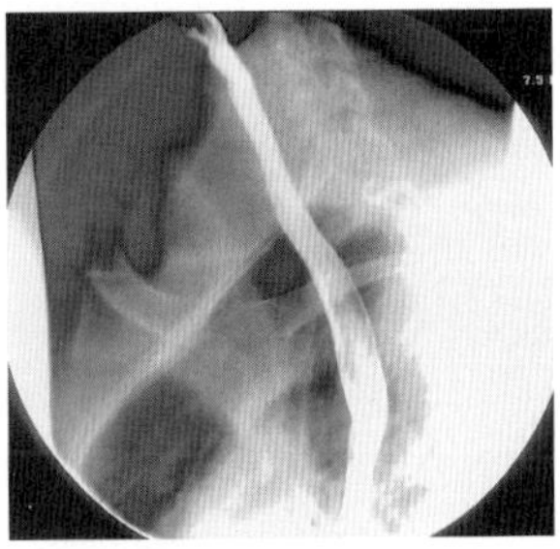

5 *Image Lateral Hypopharynx/ Cervical Esophagus*

The third swallow should focus on the hypopharynx and cervical esophagus. This last swallow requires avoiding the soft tissue mass of the left shoulder, which should be obliqued posteriorly 30°.

TABLETOP

Vertical

PATIENT

Rt Lat

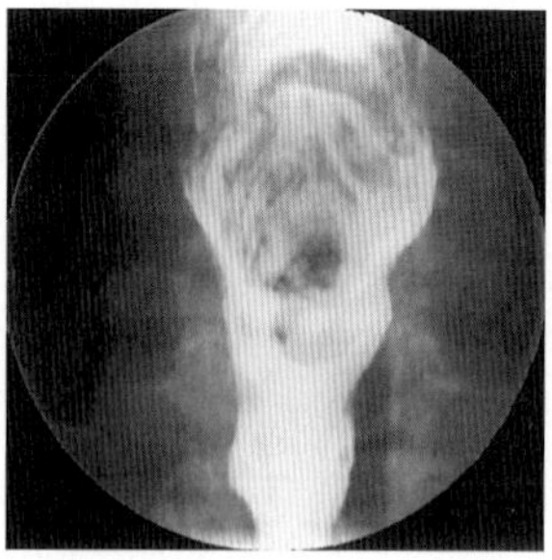

6 *Image AP Mouth/Pharynx*

Finish the exam in the AP projection. Position the collimators slightly wider than the cervical spine. The final swallow should focus on the mouth and pharynx. One swallow is usually all that is needed in this projection.

TABLETOP
Horizontal

PATIENT
AP

7 *Obtain Single Contrast Esophagram*

(see p. 22)

When the swallowing exam is normal, as is often the case, a single contrast esophagram should be obtained to find other causes of dysphagia, such as dysmotility, an esophageal stricture, or a hiatal hernia. ■

Speech Pathology Swallowing Exam

INDICATIONS

- Dysphagia (difficulty swallowing)
- Suspected aspiration

CONTRAINDICATIONS

- If pharyngeal perforation is suspected, water-soluble contrast is used by convention.
- If aspiration or a fistula to the airway is suspected, ionic water-soluble contrast is avoided.

PATIENT PREPARATION

- None

SUPPLIES

- 4 oz regular barium (60% w/v)
- 4 oz dense barium (200–250% w/v)
- Barium cup
- Liquid thickener
- Assortment of foods mixed with barium paste
- Plastic cutlery
- Suction should be available if the patient is unable to clear the airway of aspirated contents.

SCOUT FILM

- Not obtained routinely

SAMPLE DICTATION

Videofluoroscopic swallowing examination was performed in conjunction with the speech pathology department. Various liquid and solid food substances were used to assess swallowing. Normal oral transit was observed. Both regular and dense barium, as well as semisolid and solid food substances, were swallowed without difficulty. No tracheal aspiration was noted. ■

RADIATION

- Fluoro: 325 mrad/min

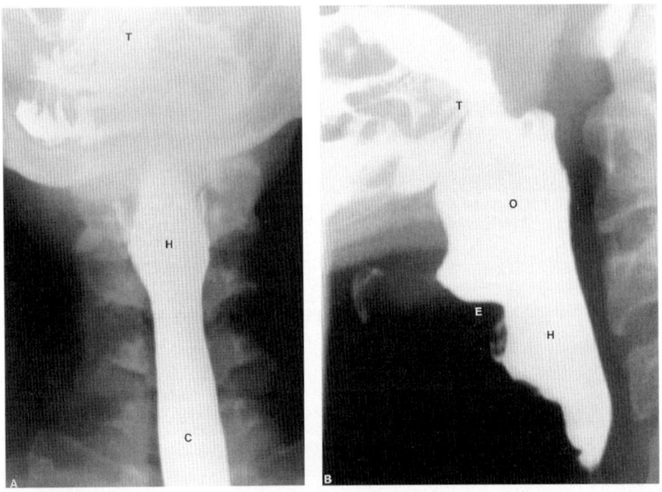

T—base of tongue
O—oropharynx
E—epiglottis
H—hypopharynx
C—cervical esophagus

FIGURE 1. *Normal anatomy of the pharynx during deglutition, as visualized in the AP (A) and lateral (B) projections. AP and lateral views of the pharynx during normal deglutition show the expected obliteration of anatomic landmarks.*

EXAM

1 Prepare Video Recorder

Record the entire exam on videotape. To coordinate imaging with the swallow, the radiologist should give the following count: "1...2...3...swallow." This allows some video recorders to come up to speed as the technologist starts recording on "1." As each swallow occurs, do not move the fluoroscope.

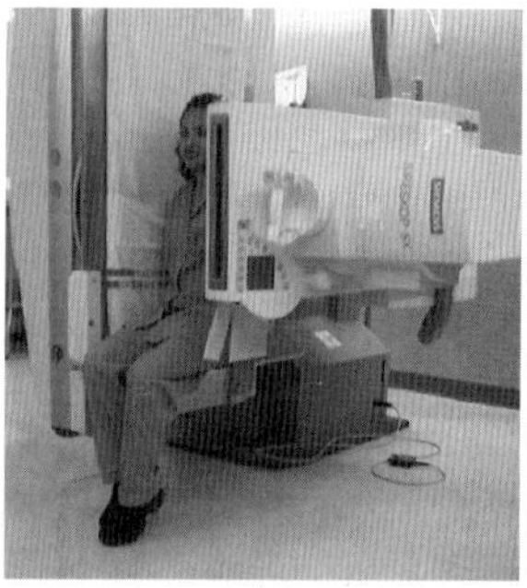

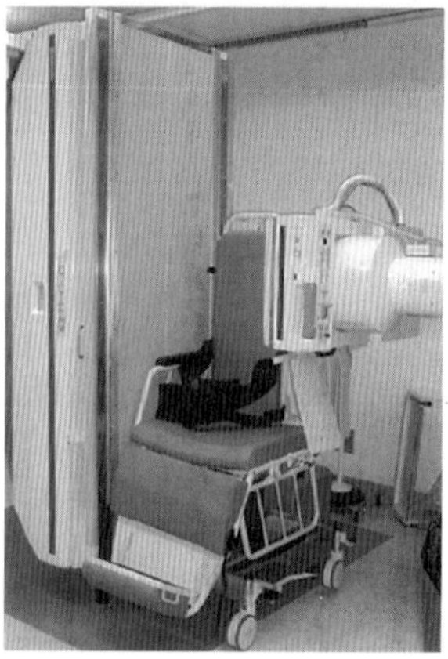

2 Position Patient

Have the patient sit on the footboard in the right lateral position, with the neck slightly extended.

Immobile patients can be placed in a fluoroscopy chair, which can be rolled into position between the tabletop and tower or secured to the footboard. If necessary, this exam can be performed with the patient in a gurney, using a C-arm fluoroscope.

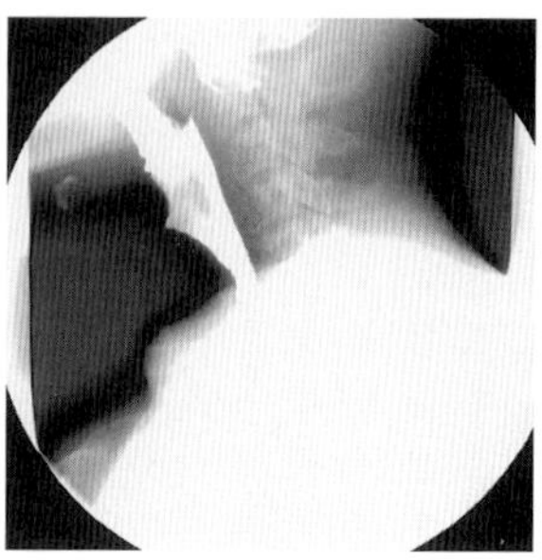

3 Record Lateral Swallow

Bring the fluoroscope into position to visualize the mouth and pharynx. The speech pathologist will administer small amounts of the designated substance to the patient. The radiologist then directs the patient to swallow. After the swallow has occurred, stop imaging.

Observe for the following findings:

1. Quality of oral transfer
2. Nasopharyngeal reflux
3. Pooling in valleculae and pyriform recesses
4. Laryngeal penetration
5. Frank tracheal aspiration (below true cords)

TABLETOP

Vertical

100–110 kVp

PATIENT

Rt Lat

3 *Record Lateral Swallow* *(continued)*

6. Cricopharyngeal achalasia (failure to relax)
7. Cricopharyngeal hypertrophy
8. Anterior osteophytosis of the cervical spine
9. Posterior pharyngeal wall thickening (edema, hematoma, abscess)

If significant aspiration occurs, terminate the exam. If the patient is unable to clear aspirated barium, suctioning may be necessary.

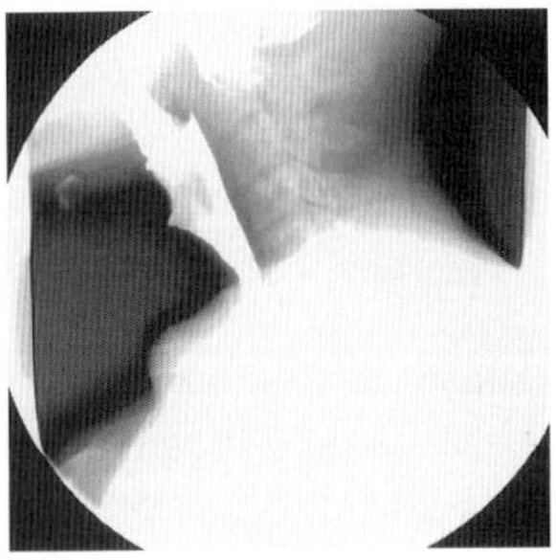

●▶

4 *Record Repeat Lateral Swallows*

The subsequent swallows follow the same sequence, except that different food substances are used. Common foods include:

1. Thinned barium
2. Thickened barium
3. Applesauce
4. Pudding
5. Cheese
6. Crackers
7. Sliced meat

TABLETOP

Vertical

PATIENT

Rt Lat

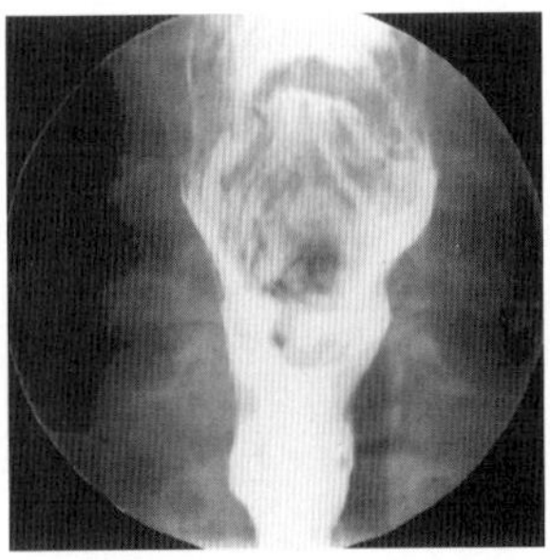

●▶

5 *Record AP Swallows*

After the lateral swallows have been completed, the patient is turned AP. Position the collimators slightly wider than the cervical spine. Observe at least one liquid barium swallow. This view should include as much of the mouth as possible and all of the pharynx.

TABLETOP

Vertical

PATIENT

AP

●▶

mag

6 *Record Phonation*

Speech pathologists occasionally wish to see the vocal cords in phonation. Simply center on the cords and use magnification while recording. ■

TABLETOP

Vertical

PATIENT

AP

Single Contrast Esophagram

INDICATIONS

- Dysphagia (difficulty swallowing)
- Odynophagia (painful swallowing)
- Globus (sensation of a lump in the throat)
- Retrosternal discomfort
- Evaluation of masses, vascular rings/slings, strictures, or aberrant anatomy
- Evaluation of esophageal motility

CONTRAINDICATIONS

- If esophageal perforation is suspected, water-soluble contrast is used by convention.

PATIENT PREPARATION

- None

SUPPLIES

- 4–6 oz regular barium (60% w/v)
- Barium cup
- Flexible large-caliber straw
- ±10 grain 13 mm diameter barium sulfate pill (e.g., E-Z-Disk, Bar-Test)
- ±2 oz regular barium (60% w/v) diluted with 2 oz water

SCOUT FILM

- Not obtained routinely

SAMPLE DICTATION

A single contrast esophagram was obtained. Normal esophageal motility was observed. There is no evidence of esophageal masses, ulcerations, strictures, or other abnormalities. No hiatal hernia is identified. ■

RADIATION

- Fluoro: 325 mrad/min
- Spot films: 10 mrad per spot film

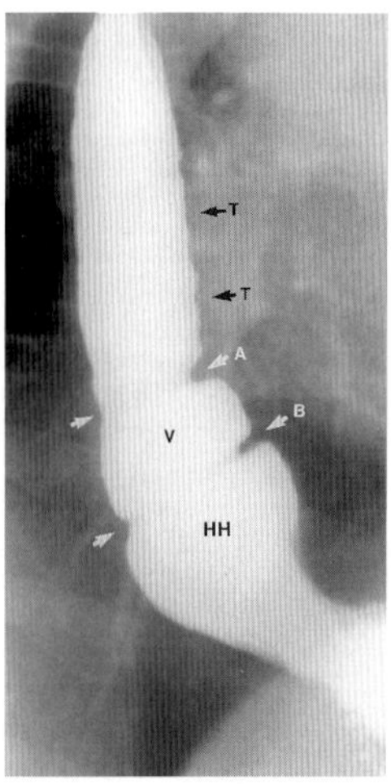

T—tertiary contraction waves (dysmotility)
A—A-ring (muscular contractile ring)
B—B-ring (mucosal ring)
V—vestibule
HH—sliding hiatal hernia

FIGURE 1. *Anatomy of the gastroesophageal junction. A mucosal ring ≥2 cm superior to the diaphragm is definitive evidence of the presence of a sliding hiatal hernia.*

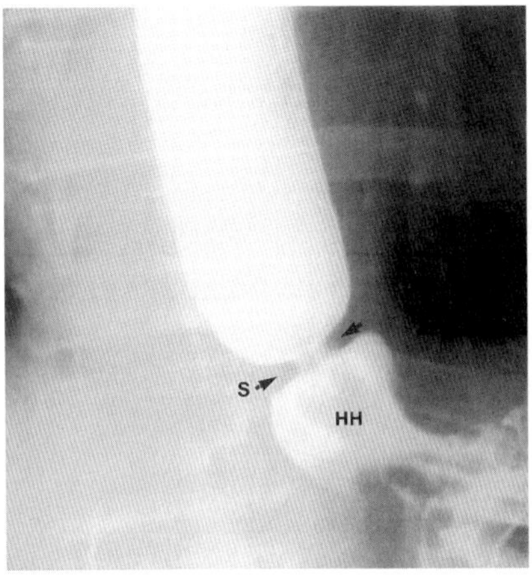

S—Schatzki ring
HH—sliding hiatal hernia

FIGURE 2. *Schatzki ring. Pathologic mucosal rings that result in dysphagia are termed Schatzki rings. Almost all rings <11 mm (and occasionally rings up to 20 mm) in diameter are symptomatic.*

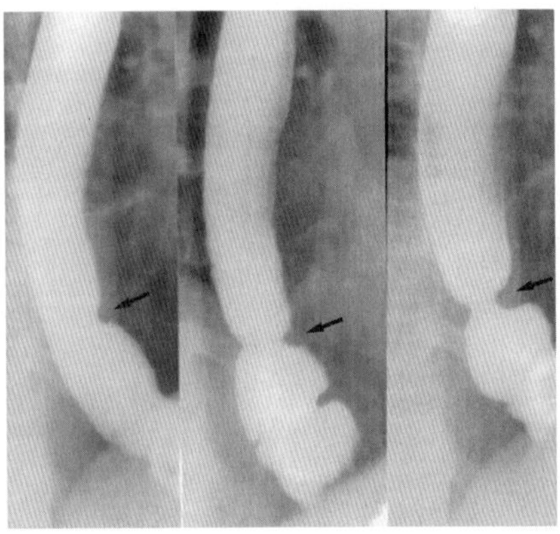

FIGURE 3. *Normal dynamic variability of the A-ring (arrows).*

EXAM

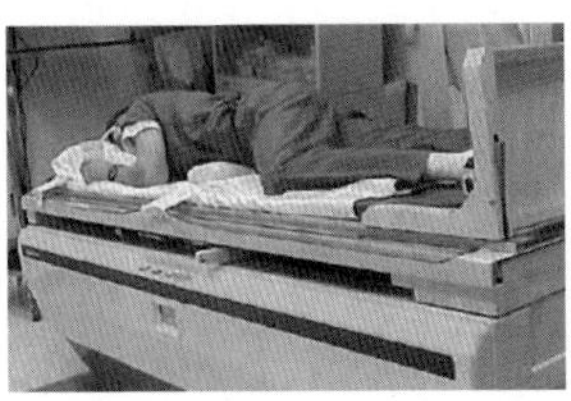

1 *Position Patient*

Place the patient in the RAO position (to offset the esophagus from the spine), with a small rectangular pad beneath the xiphoid process (to accentuate hiatal hernias by increasing intra-abdominal pressure), the right arm alongside the body, and the left knee flexed. The cup of barium should be placed by the technologist in the patient's left hand, with the straw between the teeth. The neck is turned to the left, and the head is placed flat on a pillow. Patients who are unable to tolerate this positioning may be imaged in the LPO position.

↓

TABLETOP

Head Down
−20°

PATIENT

RAO/LPO

Position Patient *(continued)*

Decline the table to −20° to allow for full esophageal distention and position the fluoroscope so that the apex of the left lung appears at the top of the monitor.

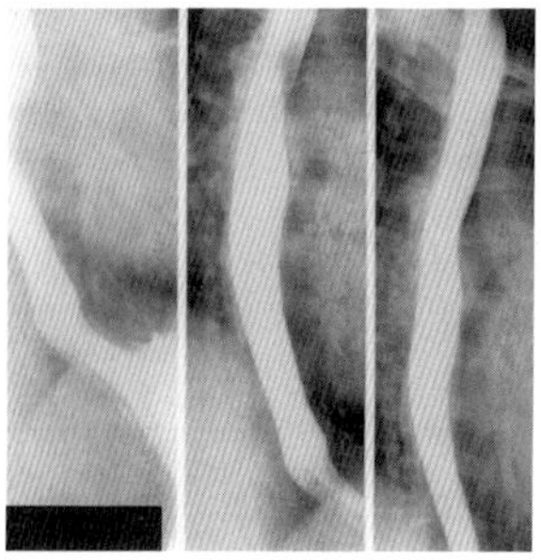

14 × 14
3 on 1
or
spot film
±mag

2 ***Image Entire Esophagus***

Have the patient continuously drink the regular barium to fill and distend the esophagus while obtaining images of:

1. The proximal esophagus
2. The midesophagus
3. The distal esophagus, including an open lower esophageal sphincter (magnified if possible)

TABLETOP
Head Down
−20°

110 kVp

PATIENT
RAO/LPO

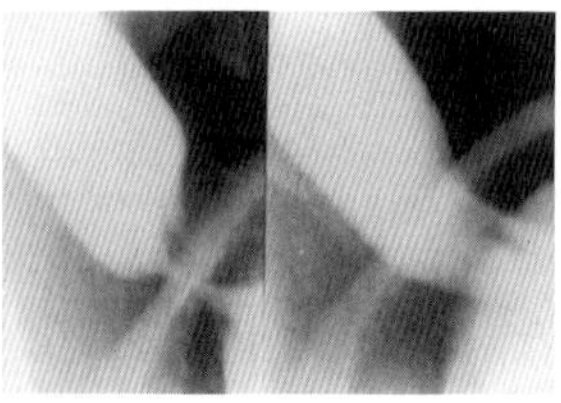

10 × 12
4 on 1
or
spot film
mag

3 ***Image Open Lower Esophageal Sphincter***

If the open lower esophageal sphincter (LES) was not captured on the prior images, it may be necessary to use rapid sequence imaging at two to four frames/sec to obtain dedicated images of this area.

Imaging an open LES avoids missing a distal esophageal stricture. ■

TABLETOP
Head Down
−20°

rapid seq
2 fr/sec

PATIENT
RAO/LPO

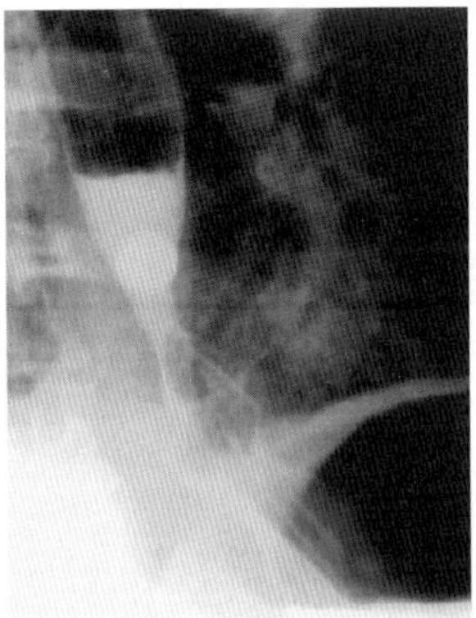

10 × 12
1 on 1
or
spot film
mag

✪ *Esophageal Stricture Evaluation*

If an esophageal stricture is identified, further characterization can be performed by attempting to pass a 13 mm barium pill through the stricture. Have the patient stand or sit on the footboard and swallow the pill followed by 2 oz regular barium diluted with 2 oz water, as undiluted barium can obscure visualization of the pill. Document the position of the pill if it cannot be passed beyond the stricture, making sure to capture the image when barium can be seen on both sides of the stricture. Calculate the width of the stricture using the following formula to compensate for magnification:

$$\text{stricture width} = \frac{(13\text{ mm})\ (\text{measured stricture on film})}{\text{measured barium pill on film}}$$

A retained pill will dissolve and pass through the gastroesophageal junction in 20–30 minutes. ■

TABLETOP
Vertical

110 kVp

PATIENT
LPO

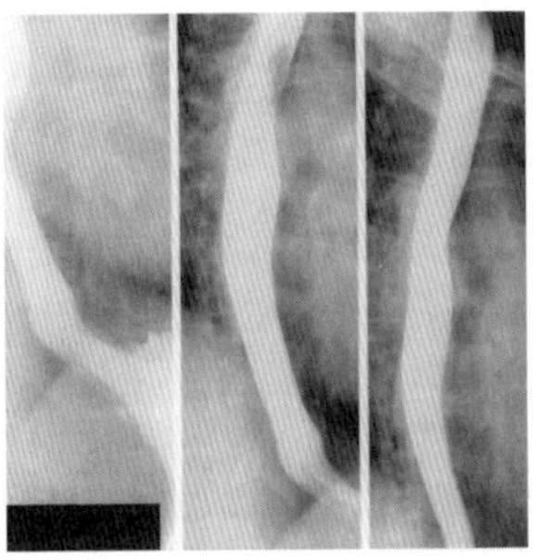

14 × 14
3 on 1
or
spot film
±mag

✪ *Single Contrast Tube Esophagram*

If the patient is unable to swallow a sufficient quantity of barium, the proximal esophagus can be intubated with an enteric feeding tube, through which contrast can be injected. Obtain images of:

1. The proximal esophagus
2. The midesophagus
3. The distal esophagus, including an open lower esophageal sphincter (magnified if possible) ■

TABLETOP
Vertical

110 kVp

PATIENT
LPO

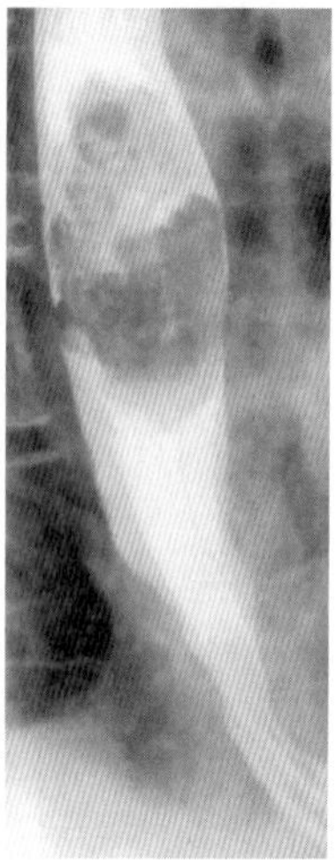

10 × 12
2 on 1
or
spot film
mag

✪ *Esophagram for Obstruction with Foreign Body*

Have the patient stand on the footboard in the LPO position to offset the esophagus from the spine. With an emesis basin accessible, have the patient swallow 2 oz dense barium. The dense barium will displace the fluid in an obstructed esophagus and outline the impacted material.

Obtain images in different obliquities to fully characterize the site of obstruction. ■

TABLETOP
Vertical

110 kVp

PATIENT
LPO
Various obliques

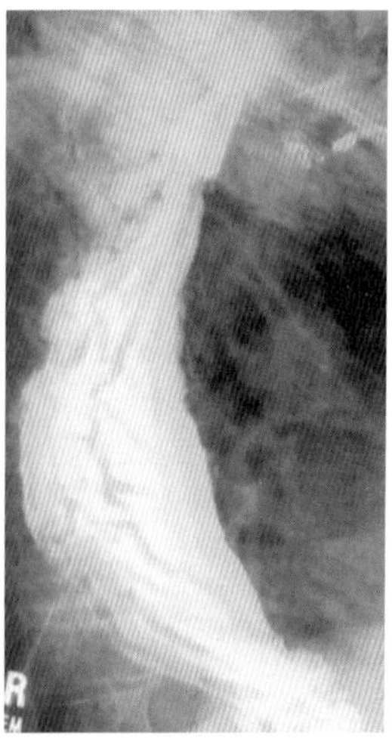

14 × 14
2 on 1
or
spot film

anastomosis
10 × 12
4 on 1
or
spot film

✪ *Gastric Pull-Through Evaluation*

Patients who have had a partial esophagogastrectomy and gastric pull-through can be imaged with single contrast technique. Beginning in the LPO position, have the patient continuously drink 6–8 oz regular barium or gastrointestinal water-soluble contrast while images are obtained of the esophagogastric anastomosis in varying obliquities. Because of rapid flooding of barium, rapid-sequence filming can be helpful. Image the entire system, including the esophageal and gastric remnants. Have the technologist obtain an overhead AP 14 × 17 film.

Early postoperative complications include leakage at the esophagogastric anastomosis and obstruction (from edema, spasm, or hematoma). Late complications include anastomotic strictures, gastroesophageal reflux, and recurrent tumor. ■

TABLETOP
Head Up
20°

110 kVp

PATIENT
LPO
Various obliques
AP

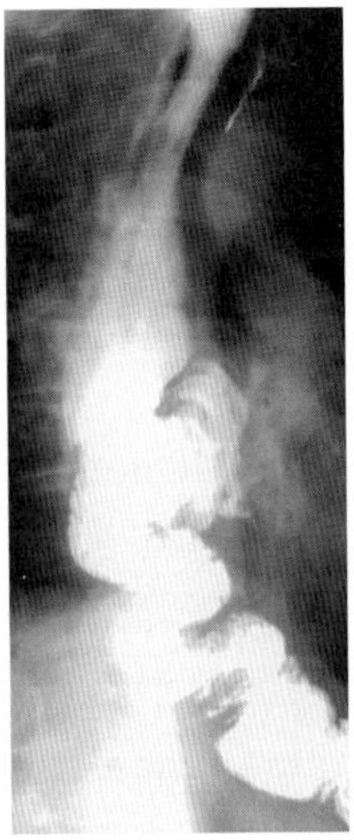

14 × 14
3 on 1
or
spot film

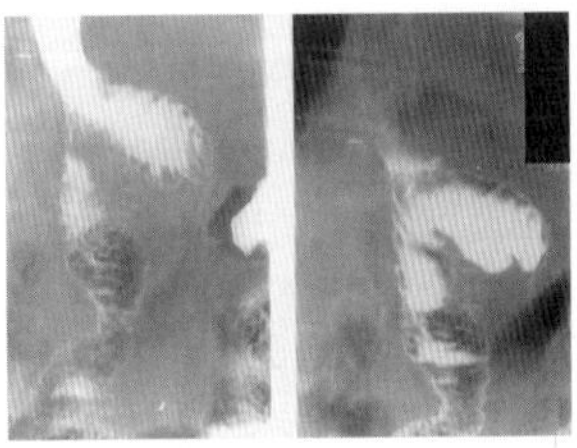

10 × 12
2 on 1
or
spot film
mag

✪ *Esophagojejunal Anastomosis Evaluation*

Patients who have had an esophagogastrectomy and jejunal pull-through can be imaged with single contrast technique. Beginning in the LPO position, have the patient continuously drink 6 oz regular barium or water-soluble contrast while images are obtained of the esophageal remnant, esophagojejunal anastomosis, and proximal small bowel. Image the anastomosis in varying obliquities. Because of rapid flooding of barium, rapid-sequence filming can be helpful. Image the entire system, including the esophageal remnant. Have the technologist obtain an overhead AP 14 × 17 film.

Early postoperative complications include leakage at the esophagojejunal anastomosis and obstruction (from edema, spasm, or hematoma). Late complications include anastomotic strictures and recurrent tumor. ■

TABLETOP
Horizontal

110 kVp

PATIENT
LPO
Various obliques
AP

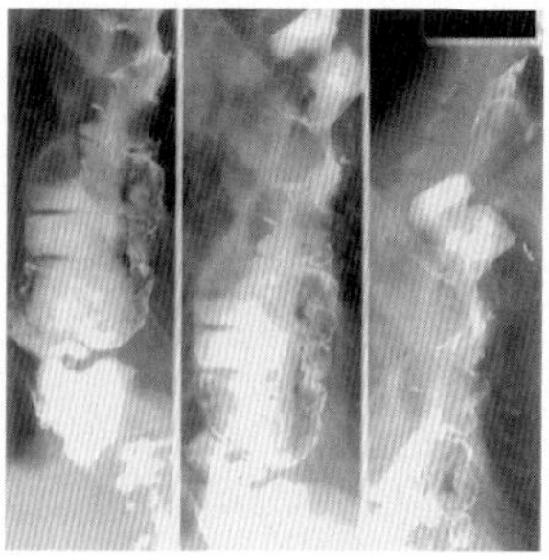

14 × 14
3 on 1
or
spot film

anastomoses
10 × 12
2–4 on 1
or
spot film
mag

✪ *Colonic Interposition Evaluation*

Patients who have had a colonic interposition can be imaged with single contrast technique. Beginning in the LPO position, have the patient continuously drink 6–8 oz regular barium or water-soluble contrast while images are obtained in various obliquities of the interposition, particularly the proximal esophagocolic and distal cologastric anastomoses. Because of rapid flooding of barium, rapid-sequence filming can be helpful. Obtain an image of the graft in the left lateral position. Have the technologist obtain an overhead AP 14 × 17 film.

Early postoperative leaks most commonly occur at the proximal anastomosis. Delayed complications include anastomotic strictures, diverticulitis, and carcinoma of the graft. ■

TABLETOP
Horizontal

110 kVp

PATIENT
LPO
Various obliques
Lt Lat
AP

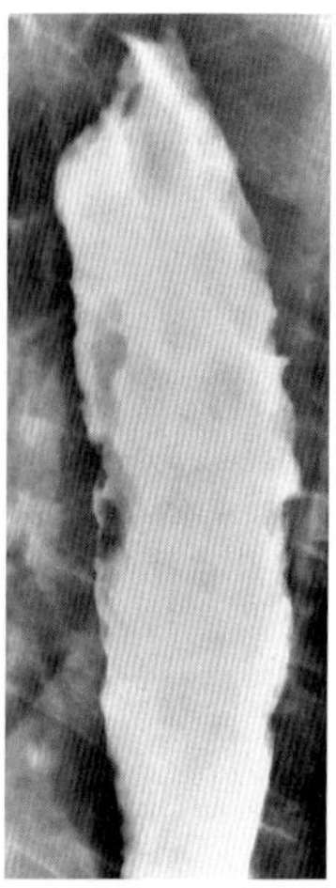

14 × 14
3 on 1
or
spot film

✪ *Esophageal Varices Evaluation*

Patients with suspected or known esophageal varices can be imaged with either single contrast technique or mucosal relief technique. Mucosal relief technique involves having the patient drink dense barium (200–250% w/v) or swallow esophageal paste, followed by imaging of the collapsed esophagus between peristaltic waves. Double contrast technique risks effacing the varices by esophageal distention.

Because esophagography can be an unreliable technique for assessing esophageal varices, endoscopy is often preferred. ■

TABLETOP
Head Down
−20°

110 kVp

PATIENT
RAO/LPO

Double Contrast Esophagram

INDICATIONS

- Early mucosal disease (erosions, polyps, tumors, inflammation, infection)

CONTRAINDICATIONS

- Suspected esophageal perforation
- Suspected aspiration
- Suspected tracheoesophageal fistula, esophageal strictures, or rings
- Evaluation of esophageal motility

PATIENT PREPARATION

- None

SUPPLIES

- 2 medicine cups (for effervescent granules and water)
- 3/4 ampule effervescent granules (e.g., Baros)
- 10 cc water
- 4–6 oz dense barium (200–250% w/v)
- Barium cup

SCOUT FILM

- Not obtained routinely

SAMPLE DICTATION

A double contrast esophagram was obtained using dense barium. The esophageal mucosa has a normal appearance. There is no evidence of ulcerations, masses, strictures, or other abnormalities. ■

RADIATION

- Fluoro: 325 mrad/min
- Spot films: 10 mrad per spot film

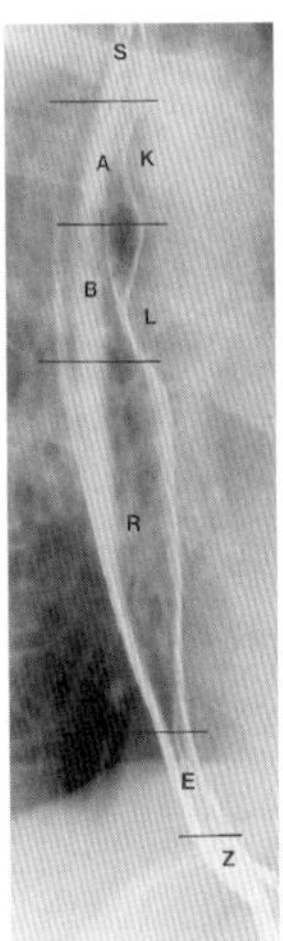

K—aortic knob impression
L—left mainstem bronchial impression
S—supra-aortic segment (from thoracic inlet to superior aspect of the aortic arch)
A—aortic arch segment (through aortic arch to carina)
B—bronchial segment (from carina through left mainstem bronchus)
R—retrocardiac segment (from left mainstem bronchus to left lateral deviation)
E—epiphrenic segment (from left lateral deviation to esophageal hiatus)
Z—sphincter zone (from esophageal hiatus to gastroesophageal junction)

FIGURE 1. *Normal anatomy of the esophagus.*

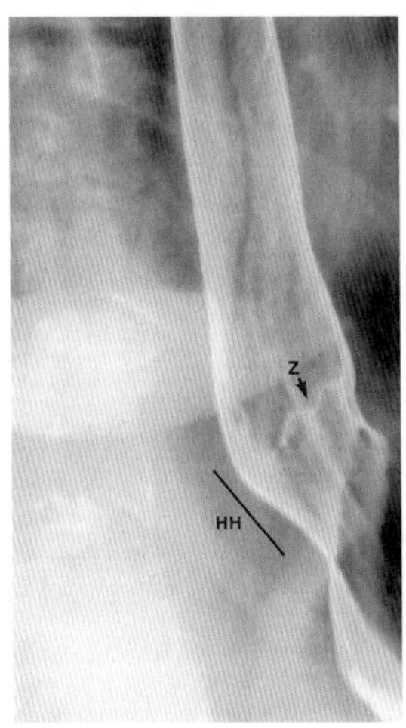

Z—Z-line (squamosal-columnar mucosal junction)
HH—hiatal hernia (from Z-line to diaphragm)

FIGURE 2. *Anatomy of the gastroesophageal junction.*

EXAM

1 *Position Patient*

Have the patient stand on the footboard in the LPO position (to offset the esophagus from the spine). Place the cup of dense barium in the patient's left hand. Have the patient take a small sip of the dense barium to become acclimated to its consistency. If the patient appears unable to tolerate the dense barium, obtain a single contrast esophagram.

TABLETOP
Vertical

PATIENT
LPO

2 *Instruct Patient on Swallowing Sequence*

Explain the following sequence to the patient until understanding is demonstrated, as strict patient cooperation is essential for obtaining a satisfactory exam:

1. The patient's head is tilted back by extending the neck.
2. The radiologist pours the granules into the back of the mouth.
3. The radiologist pours the water into the mouth.
4. The patient immediately swallows the granules and water.
5. The patient drinks the barium, one swallow after another with moderate rapidity and with constant encouragement by the radiologist.
6. Caution the patient not to burp.

TABLETOP
Vertical

PATIENT
LPO

3 *Position Fluoroscope*

Center the fluoroscope over the upper third of the esophagus to localize the esophagus; then lower the tower and administer the effervescent granules and water as directed above. Using only 3/4 ampule of the effervescent granules prevents overdistention with gas.

TABLETOP
Vertical

PATIENT
LPO

4 *Image Entire Esophagus*

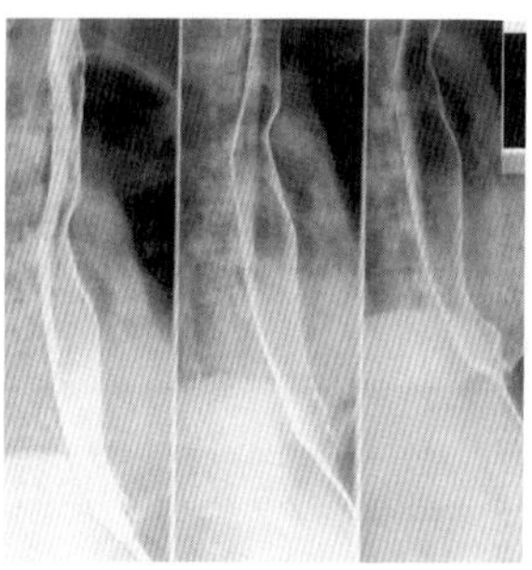

14 × 14
3 on 1
or
spot film

As the patient is drinking, observe the esophagus for a "silver-satin" appearance, indicating the best possible coating, and obtain images of:

1. The proximal esophagus
2. The midesophagus
3. The distal esophagus

If the patient cannot retain the air from the effervescent granules, abort the exam and obtain a single contrast esophagram. ■

TABLETOP
Vertical

90 kVp

PATIENT
LPO

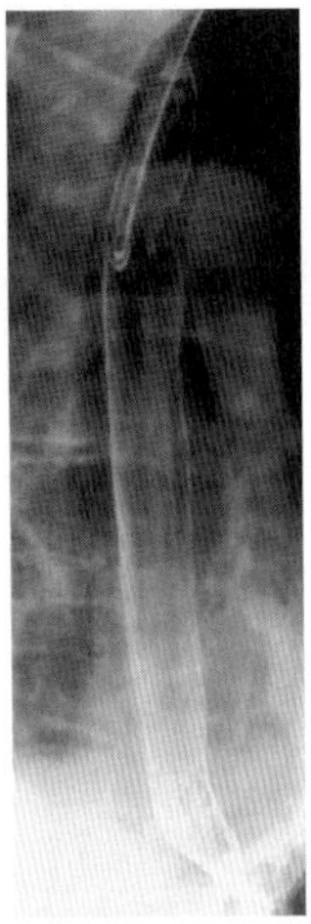

14 × 14
1–3 on 1
or
spot film

✪ *Double Contrast Tube Esophagram*

A double contrast tube esophagram is a rarely encountered exam. It is obtained in patients who are unable to swallow a sufficient quantity of dense barium or effervescent granules. A red rubber catheter is inserted through the nose and placed in the proximal esophagus. Then 4 oz of dense barium (200–250% w/v) are swallowed by mouth while air is gently insufflated into the esophagus with a pneumatic bulb and images of the entire esophagus are obtained.

TABLETOP
Head Up
30°

90 kVp

PATIENT
LPO

Esophagram for Perforation

INDICATIONS

- Suspected esophageal perforation

CONTRAINDICATIONS

- Ionic water-soluble contrast is contraindicated in patients who may aspirate.

PATIENT PREPARATION

- None

SUPPLIES

- 4–6 oz chilled 37% iodine gastrointestinal water-soluble contrast (e.g., Gastrografin, MD-Gastroview)
- 4–6 oz regular barium (60% w/v)
- Barium cup
- Large-caliber, flexible straw

SCOUT FILM

- PA/lateral chest

SAMPLE DICTATION

A single contrast esophagram was obtained to evaluate for esophageal perforation. The exam was initially performed using Gastrografin, followed with regular barium after no gross leakage was identified. There was no evidence of extravasation of contrast or other significant abnormality. ■

RADIATION

- Fluoro: 325 mrad/min
- Spot films: 10 mrad per spot film

EXAM

1 *Position Patient*

Place the patient in the LPO position, using a triangular foam pad against the back.

If the patient is too ill to drink contrast, it may be necessary to place a tube in the proximal esophagus through which contrast can be injected.

TABLETOP
Horizontal

PATIENT
LPO

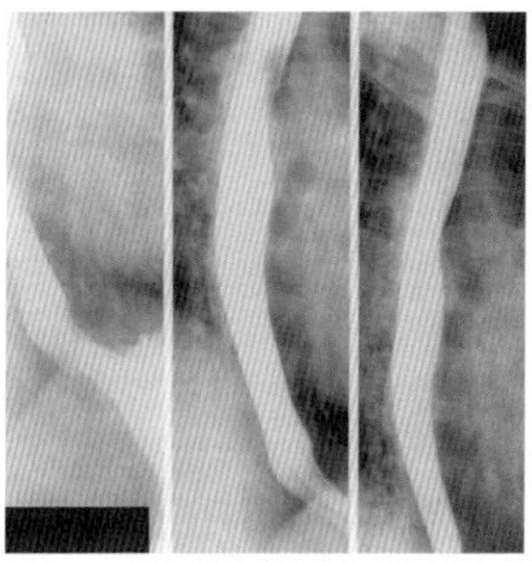

14 × 14
3 on 1
or
spot film

2 *Image Entire Esophagus (Water-Soluble Contrast)*

If there is no risk of aspiration, have the patient drink 4–6 oz water-soluble contrast (chilled to make the bitter solution more palatable) while obtaining overlapping images of:

1. The proximal esophagus
2. The midesophagus
3. The distal esophagus

TABLETOP
Horizontal

75 kVp

PATIENT
LPO

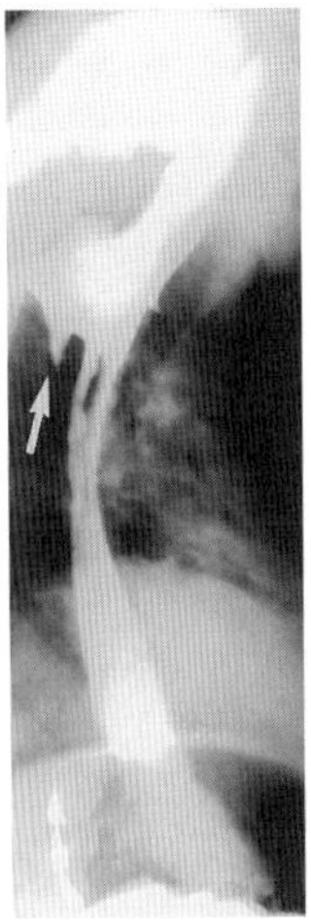

14 × 14
3 on 1
or
spot film

3 *Image Leak (if identified)*

If a leak is identified, obtain images in different obliquities to characterize it fully; then terminate the exam.

TABLETOP
Horizontal

PATIENT
Various obliques

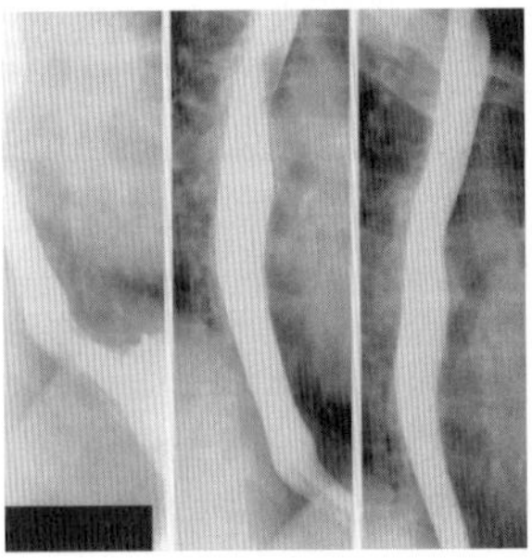

14 × 14
3 on 1
or
spot film

4 *Image Entire Esophagus (Barium)*

If there is no evidence of leakage of water-soluble contrast or if there is a risk of the patient aspirating (prohibiting use of water-soluble contrast), continue the exam using barium. Because barium is denser than water-soluble contrast, it will show smaller areas of leakage. Have the patient drink 4–6 oz of regular barium while obtaining overlapping images of:

1. The upper esophagus
2. The midesophagus
3. The lower esophagus

TABLETOP
Horizontal

110 kVp

PATIENT
LPO

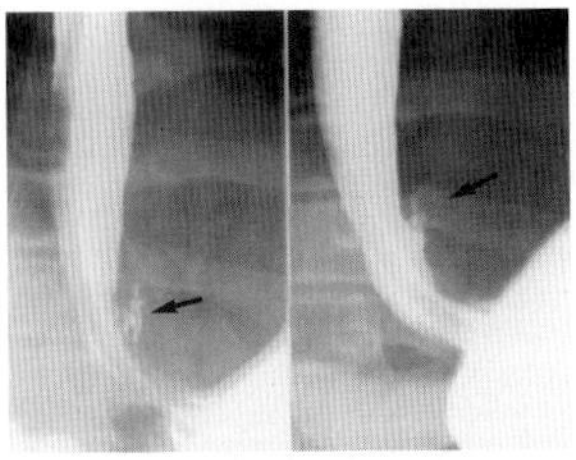

14 × 14
2–3 on 1
or
spot film

5 *Image Leak (if identified)*

If a leak is identified, obtain images in different obliquities to fully characterize it. ■

TABLETOP
Horizontal

PATIENT
Various obliques

PART II

Upper Gastrointestinal Examinations

Michael Davis, M.D.
Jeffrey D. Houston, M.D.

Single Contrast Upper Gastrointestinal Series

Single Contrast Upper Gastrointestinal Series with Small Bowel Follow-Through

Biphasic Upper Gastrointestinal Series

Fundoplication Evaluation

Vertical Gastric Banding Evaluation

Billroth Evaluation

Enteric Feeding Tube Placement

Double Contrast Enteroclysis

Single Contrast Upper Gastrointestinal Series

INDICATIONS

- To precede a small bowel series
- Inability to tolerate biphasic upper gastrointestinal (UGI) series (nausea, vomiting, decreased mobility)
- Assessment of gastric peristalsis or for gastric outlet obstruction
- Suspected hiatal hernia
- Evaluation of masses, varices, strictures, fistulas, or aberrant anatomy
- Postpyloroplasty

CONTRAINDICATIONS

- If perforation is suspected, water-soluble contrast is used by convention.

PATIENT PREPARATION

- NPO after midnight or 6 hours prior to exam

SUPPLIES

- 2 oz, then 4–6 oz regular barium (60% w/v)
- Barium cup
- Large-caliber flexible straw

SCOUT FILM

- Not obtained routinely

SAMPLE DICTATION

Normal esophageal motility was observed. The esophagus has a normal appearance. The gastric folds appear normal. No gastric masses, scars, or other abnormalities are identified. All portions of the duodenum and the visualized proximal jejunum appear normal. ■

RADIATION

- Fluoro: 650 mrad/min
- Spot films: 50 mrad per spot film

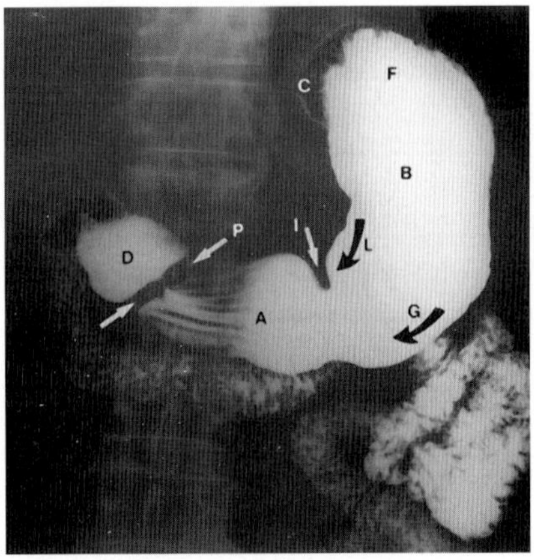

F—fundus
C—cardia
B—body (corpus)
A—antrum (pyloric antrum)
P—pylorus (pyloric canal)
D—duodenal bulb
L—lesser curvature
G—greater curvature
I—angular notch (incisura angularis)

FIGURE 1. *Normal gastric anatomy.*

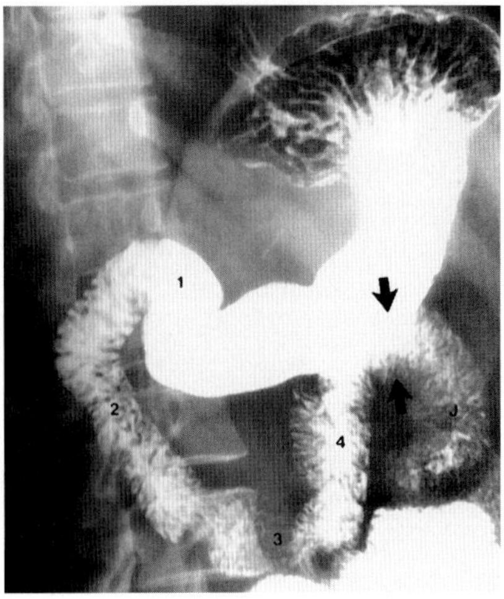

1—first portion of duodenum (duodenal bulb)

2—second (descending) portion of duodenum

3—third (transverse) portion of duodenum

4—fourth (ascending) portion of duodenum

arrows—duodenojejunal junction (at attachment of ligament of Treitz)

J—jejunum

FIGURE 2. *Normal duodenal anatomy.*

EXAM

1 *Scan Esophagus*

Position the fluoroscope so that the apex of the left lung appears at the top of the monitor. Have the patient drink 2 oz regular barium (60% w/v) and quickly scan the esophagus from the pharynx to the lower esophageal sphincter.

TABLETOP
Vertical

110 kVp

PATIENT
LPO

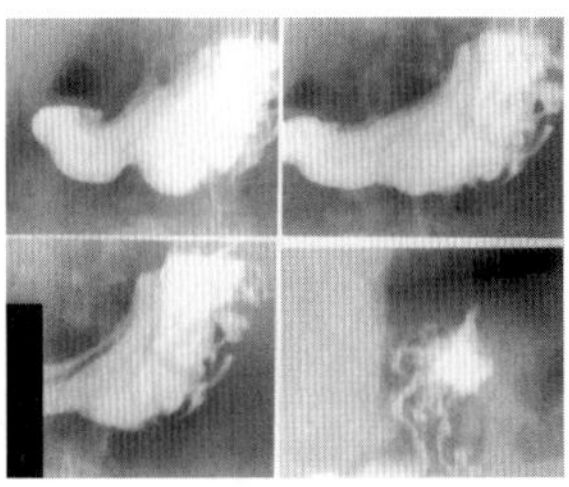

10 × 12
4 on 1
or
spot film
mag

2 *Image Stomach with Compression*

Compress the gastric antrum and body against the spine with a compression cone or paddle to reveal the gastric folds, keeping the spine in the center of the field as you rotate the patient. If the folds are difficult to see, decline the table to 45° and compress again. The superior body and fundus are under the ribs and cannot be compressed. Bring the table to the horizontal position to image the fundus.

TABLETOP
Vertical

PATIENT
LPO → RPO
AP

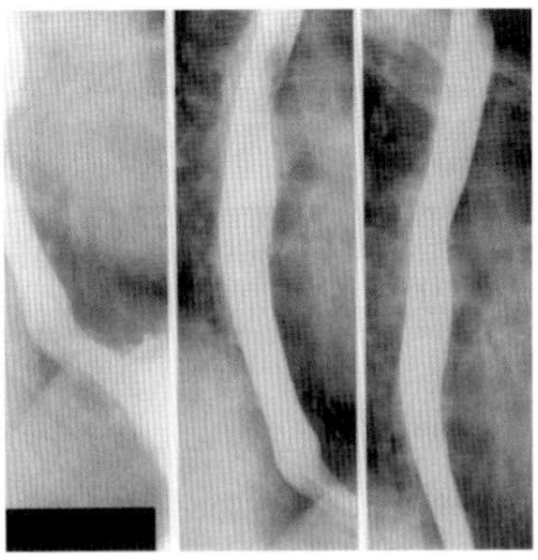

14 × 14
3 on 1
or
spot film
±mag

3 *Obtain Single Contrast Esophagram*

(see p. 22)

Position the fluoroscope so that the apex of the left lung appears at the top of the screen. Have the patient drink 4–6 oz regular barium (60% w/v) to fill and distend the esophagus, and obtain images of:

1. The proximal esophagus
2. The midesophagus
3. The distal esophagus, including an open lower esophageal sphincter (magnified if possible)

TABLETOP
Head Down
−20°

PATIENT
RAO

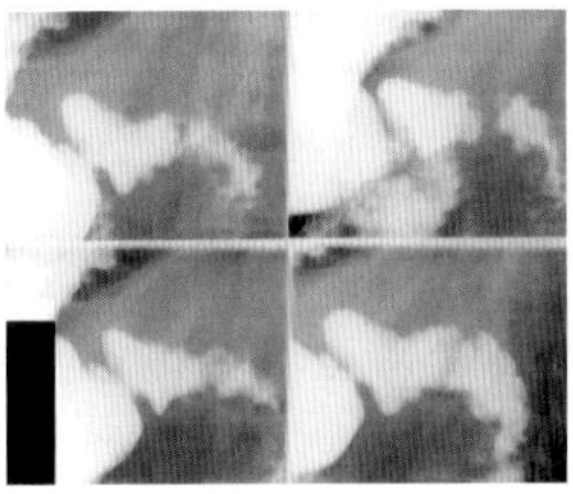

10 × 12
4 on 1
or
spot film
mag

4 *Image Duodenal Bulb*

Visualize the barium-filled duodenal bulb and obtain at least four slightly different views. If the bulb is not well seen, have the patient inhale deeply and stop breathing briefly to improve visualization of the bulb.

Alternatively, the patient can be placed prone and the duodenal bulb can be compressed from underneath by using a balloon compression paddle.

TABLETOP
Horizontal

PATIENT
Rt Lat
±PA

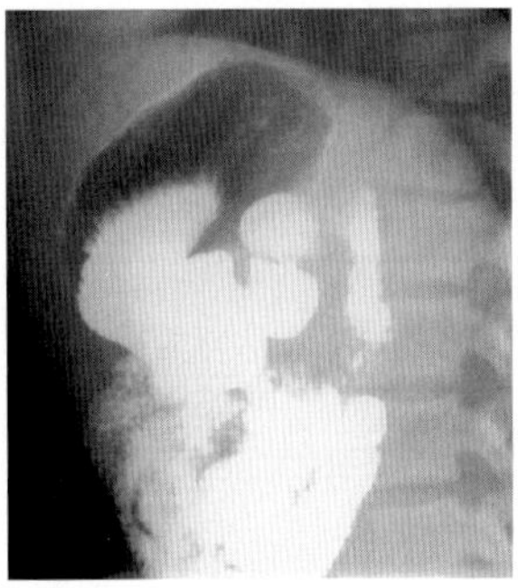

14 × 14
1 on 1

5 *Image Right Lateral Stomach*

Image the stomach and duodenal bulb in the right lateral or RAO position, centering these structures on the image.

Alternatively, the technologist can obtain this image as an overhead film.

TABLETOP
Horizontal

PATIENT
Rt Lat/RAO

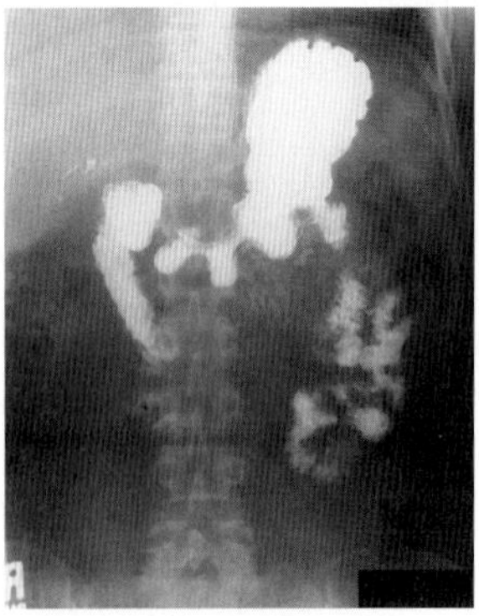

14 × 17

6 *Obtain Overhead Film(s)*

Have the technologist obtain an overhead PA film. The stomach should be positioned at the superior aspect of the film, so as to visualize as much of the proximal small bowel as possible. ■

TABLETOP

Horizontal

90 kVp

PATIENT

PA

Single Contrast Upper Gastrointestinal Series with Small Bowel Follow-Through

INDICATIONS

- Evaluation of small bowel obstruction
- Malabsorption, diarrhea
- Systemic diseases such as progressive systemic sclerosis (scleroderma), celiac disease, hypoproteinemia
- Gastrointestinal bleeding, anemia of unknown origin

CONTRAINDICATIONS

- If perforation is suspected, water-soluble contrast is used by convention.

PATIENT PREPARATION

- NPO after midnight or 6 hours prior to exam

SUPPLIES

- 2 oz, then 4–6 oz regular barium (60% w/v) (for single contrast UGI series)
- 8–10 oz regular barium (60% w/v) (for small bowel series)
- Barium cup
- Large-caliber flexible straw
- 10 mg (2 cc) metoclopramide
- 3 cc syringe (for metoclopramide)
- 18 gauge needle (for drawing metoclopramide)
- 25 gauge needle (for injecting metoclopramide)
- Tourniquet
- Alcohol swab
- Small bandage

SCOUT FILM

- AP abdomen

SAMPLE DICTATION

A single contrast upper gastrointestinal series was initially performed. Normal esophageal motility was observed. The esophagus, stomach, and duodenum have a normal appearance. After the intravenous administration of 10 mg metoclopramide, a small bowel series was performed. The mucosal folds throughout the jejunum and ileum appear normal. No strictures, masses, or other small bowel abnormalities are identified. Normal small bowel transit was observed. The terminal ileum was well visualized with compression and is unremarkable. ■

RADIATION

- Fluoro: 1000 mrad/min
- Spot films: 50 mrad per spot film

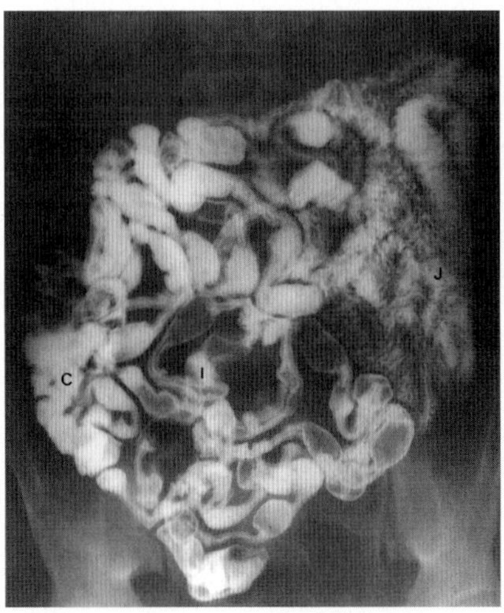

J—jejunum
I—ileum
C—cecum

FIGURE 1. *Normal small bowel anatomy.*

EXAM

1 *Perform Single Contrast UGI* *(see p. 37)*

Perform a routine single contrast UGI series.

℞

2 *Administer Metoclopramide*

If not contraindicated, administer 10 mg metoclopramide (intravenously if possible) over 1–2 minutes, as a rapid bolus can result in a feeling of anxiety followed by drowsiness. Metoclopramide increases peristalsis, resulting in a significantly quicker exam.

TABLETOP
Head Up
20–30°

PATIENT
AP

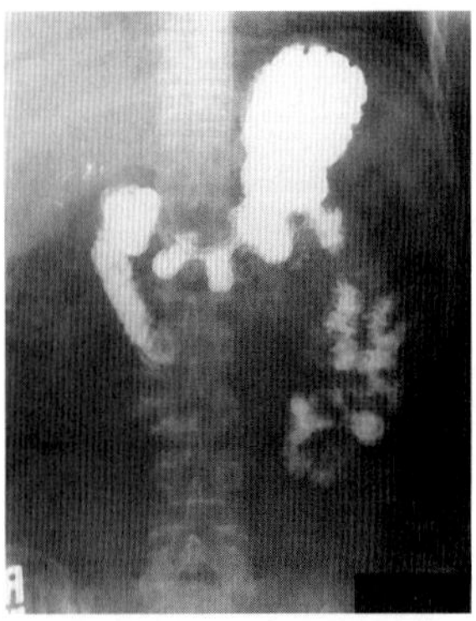

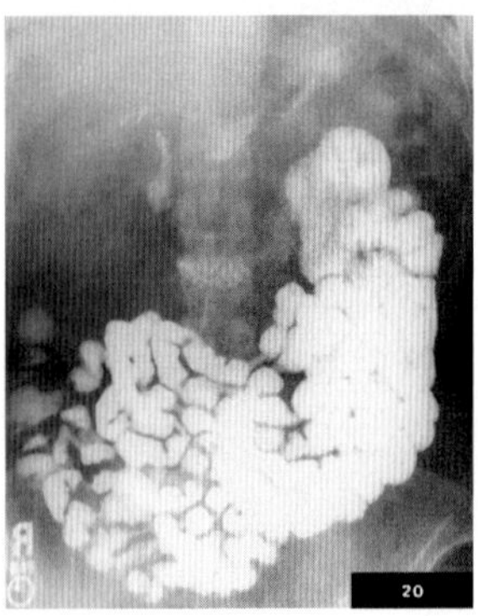

14 × 17

3 *Obtain Sequential Overhead Films*

Have the patient drink 8–10 oz additional regular barium. Have the technologist obtain overhead PA abdominal films at 20 minute intervals (or longer if indicated) until barium reaches the cecum or ascending colon.

It may be necessary to have the patient drink additional barium periodically to keep the stomach and proximal small bowel opacified.

TABLETOP
Horizontal

90 kVp

PATIENT
PA

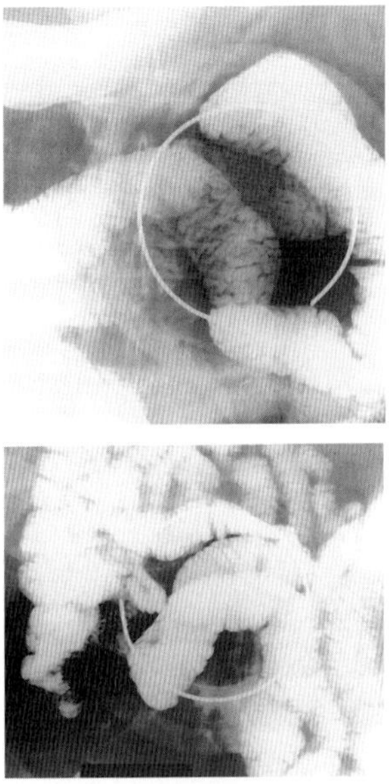

10 × 12
1 on 1
or
spot film

4 *Obtain Spot Films of Jejunum and Ileum*

When the jejunum and ileum are well visualized, obtain one or two AP spot films of each, using the compression cone or balloon paddle to separate the loops.

Using a lead glove to separate the loops, fluoroscopically inspect all the bowel loops, looking for abnormalities.

If the terminal ileum becomes filled but barium will not advance into the cecum in a timely fashion, the patient can drink 4 oz chilled water to stimulate peristalsis.

TABLETOP
Horizontal

90 kVp

PATIENT
AP

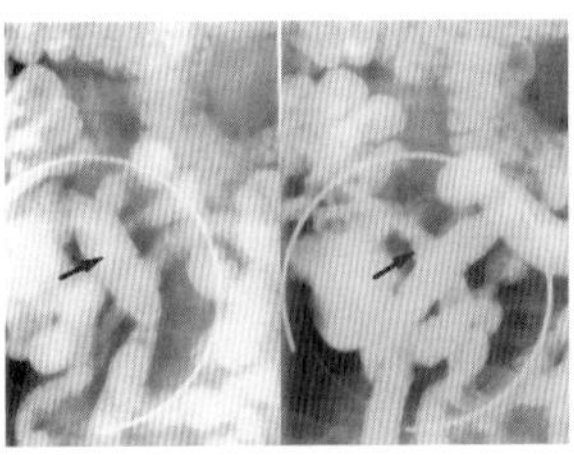

10 × 12
2–3 on 1
or
spot film

5 *Image Terminal Ileum*

After barium is visualized in the cecum or ascending colon on the overhead films, obtain two or three compression views of the ileocecal valve and the terminal ileum.

The ileocecal valve and the terminal ileum can be seen best in most patients by turning them slightly LPO and compressing. The occasional posterior ileocecal valve requires that the patient be turned RPO. ■

TABLETOP
Horizontal

PATIENT
LPO/RPO

Biphasic Upper Gastrointestinal Series

INDICATIONS

- Mucosal disease (early erosions, ulcerations, polyps, cancer)

CONTRAINDICATIONS

- Suspected perforation
- A biphasic exam should not precede a small bowel series so as not to fill the small bowel with dense barium.

PATIENT PREPARATION

- NPO after midnight or 6 hours prior to exam

SUPPLIES

- 0.2 mg glucagon
- 1 cc syringe (for glucagon)
- 18 gauge needle (for drawing glucagon)
- 25 gauge needle (for injecting glucagon)
- Tourniquet
- Alcohol swab
- Small bandage
- 2 oz, then 4–6 oz regular barium (60% w/v)
- Barium cup
- Large-caliber flexible straw
- 3/4 ampule effervescent granules (e.g., Baros)
- 10 cc water
- 2 medicine cups (for effervescent granules and water)
- 4–6 oz dense barium (200–250% w/v)

SCOUT FILM

- Not obtained routinely

SAMPLE DICTATION

Normal esophageal motility was observed. The esophagus, stomach, and proximal small bowel have a normal single contrast appearance. After the intravenous administration of 0.2 mg glucagon, a double contrast upper gastrointestinal series was performed. Examination of the esophagus, stomach, and duodenum reveals normal mucosal features in each segment. ■

RADIATION

- Fluoro: 650 mrad/min
- Spot films: 50 mrad per spot film

EXAM

℞

1 *Administer Glucagon*

If not contraindicated, administer 0.2 mg glucagon (intravenously if possible). Glucagon causes temporary paralysis of the gut, which reduces spasm and motion artifact.

TABLETOP

Head Up 20–30°

PATIENT

AP

2 *Perform Single Contrast UGI* *(see p. 37)*

Follow steps 1 through 4 for a single contrast UGI series. Do not wait for the duodenal bulb to fill with barium, as the effect of glucagon rapidly diminishes.

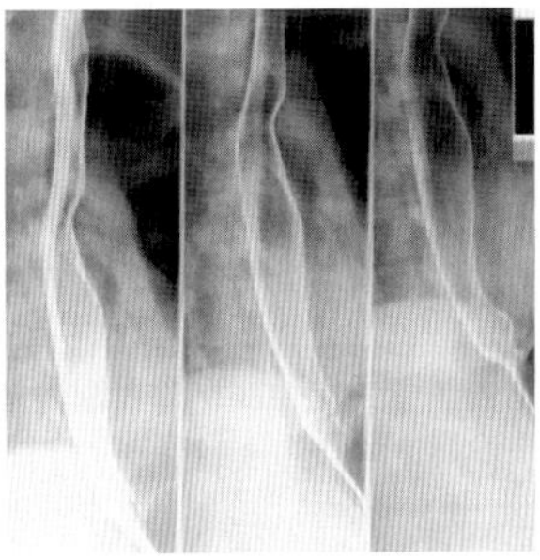

14 × 14
3 on 1
or
spot film

3 *Obtain Double Contrast Esophagram*
(see p. 29)

Pour the effervescent granules and 10 cc water into the patient's mouth. Have the patient swallow and then quickly drink 4 oz dense barium. Caution the patient not to burp.

As the patient is drinking, observe the esophagus for a "silver-satin" appearance, indicating the best possible coating, and obtain images of:

1. The proximal esophagus
2. The midesophagus
3. The distal esophagus

TABLETOP
Vertical

90 kVp

PATIENT
LPO

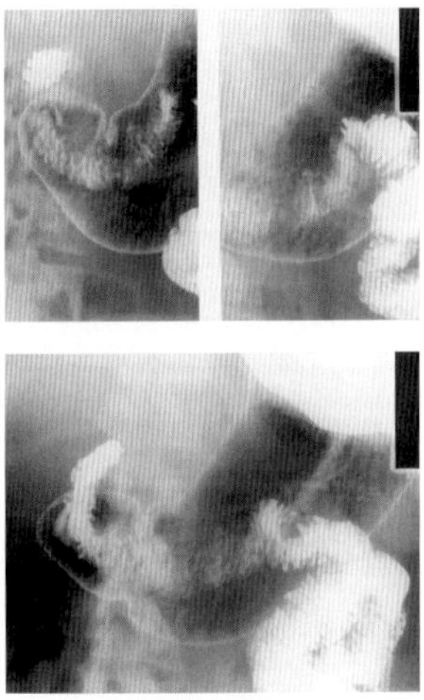

10 × 12
1–2 on 1
or
spot film

4 *Image Gastric Antrum and Body*

Decline the table to horizontal, roll the patient to the prone position, and rock the hips from side to side 8–10 times to optimize mucosal coating. Pull the patient from prone to LPO to film the antrum, then AP to film the antrum and body. Take several slightly different views of these areas.

TABLETOP
Horizontal

PATIENT
LPO
AP

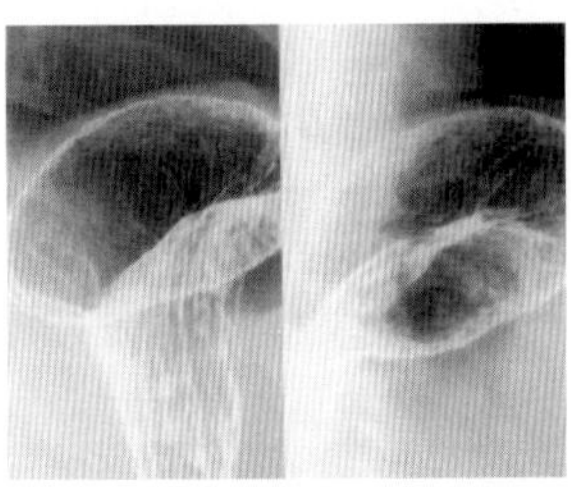

10 × 12
2 on 1
or
spot film

5 *Image Gastric Fundus*

Turn the patient to the right lateral position and film the fundus, or bring the tabletop to the vertical position and film the fundus in AP and LPO projections.

It may be necessary to have the patient retract overlying breast tissue to avoid unnecessary irradiation and image degradation.

TABLETOP
Horizontal
±Vertical

PATIENT
Rt Lat
±AP/LPO

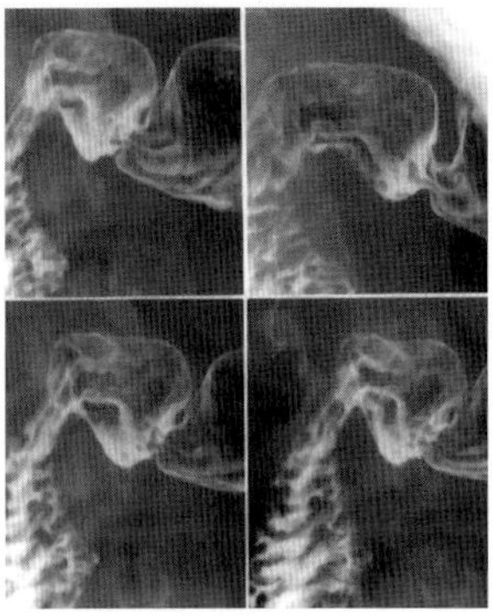

10 × 12
4 on 1
or
spot film
mag

6a *Image Duodenal Bulb*

Keep the patient in the right lateral position until the duodenal bulb fills with dense barium; then turn the patient to the left lateral position. When gas fills the bulb, take several representative images in varying obliquities.

TABLETOP

Horizontal

PATIENT

Rt Lat → Lt Lat

Various obliques

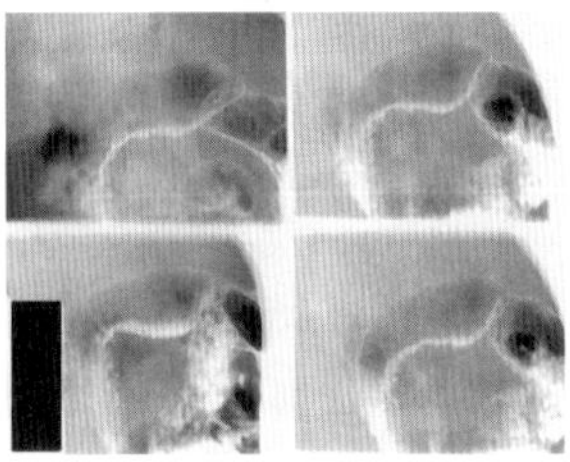

10 × 12
4–6 on 1
or
spot film
mag

6b *Image Duodenal Bulb (Alternative)*

If the above technique is unsuccessful, a longer alternative method can be attempted to image the duodenal bulb. With the patient in the right lateral position and the bulb filled with dense barium, place the patient prone. Wait a few seconds, then have the patient roll away from you 360° until prone again. Raise the table upright to 70° and rotate the patient into the LPO or AP position (whichever shows the bulb best) and image the gas-filled bulb.

If the bulb does not fill in 1–1½ minutes, leave the room for 3–5 minutes before attempting the procedure again.

TABLETOP

Various

PATIENT

PA → PA

LPO/AP

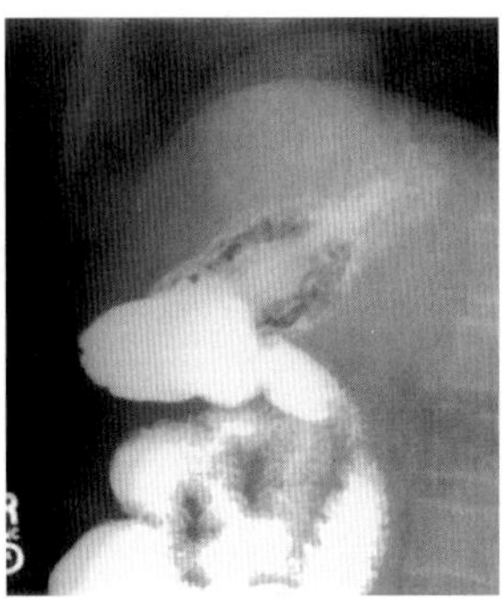

14 × 14

7 *Image Right Lateral Stomach*

With the table horizontal, turn the patient to the right lateral position and image the stomach, which should be centered on the film. Alternatively, the technologist can obtain this image as an overhead film.

TABLETOP

Horizontal

110 kVp

PATIENT

Rt Lat

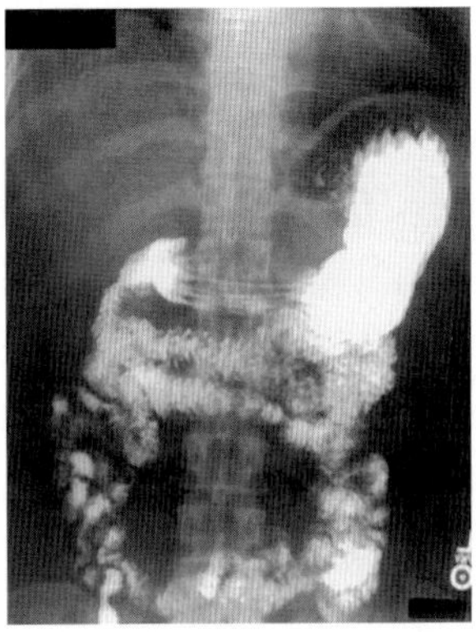

14 × 17

8 *Obtain Overhead Film*

Have the technologist obtain an overhead film that includes the stomach, duodenum, and two or more loops of jejunum. The exam is not complete until at least two loops of jejunum are visualized. ■

TABLETOP

Horizontal

90 kVp

PATIENT

PA

Fundoplication Evaluation

INDICATIONS

- Prior fundoplication or Angelchik anti-reflux prosthesis

CONTRAINDICATIONS

- Postoperative exams to exclude leakage should be performed with water-soluble contrast

PATIENT PREPARATION

- NPO after midnight or 6 hours prior to exam

SUPPLIES

- ±4–8 oz chilled 37% iodine water-soluble gastrointestinal contrast (e.g., Gastrografin, MD-Gastroview)
- 6 oz regular barium (60% w/v)
- Barium cup
- Large-caliber flexible straw

SCOUT FILM

- AP abdomen

SAMPLE DICTATION

A limited upper gastrointestinal series was performed to evaluate the patient's recent Nissen fundoplication. As the procedure was ordered to exclude a postoperative leak, Gastrografin was initially used, followed with regular barium. The gastroesophageal junction is narrowed at the site of the fundoplication, as expected, but remains patent. No postoperative leakage of contrast is identified. ■

RADIATION

- Fluoro: 650 mrad/min
- Spot films: 50 rad per spot film

TABLE 1. *Variations of Gastric Fundoplications Employed for Gastroesophageal Reflux and Hiatal Hernia Repair*

SURGICAL PROCEDURE	DESCRIPTION
Nissen fundoplication	Reduction of hernia with 360° fundal wrap surrounding a 4 cm segment of the intra-abdominal esophagus.
Toupet fundoplication	Reduction of hernia employing a 270° posterior fundal wrap.
Belsey Mark IV repair	Reduction of hernia with restoration of a 3 cm segment of intra-abdominal esophagus using a 240° wrap around the anterior and left lateral distal esophagus.
Hill posterior gastropexy	Reduction of hernia using a ≤180° fundal wrap with suturing of the proximal lesser curvature to the median arcuate ligament.
Collis gastropexy	Gastropexy performed on patients with esophageal strictures and contraction that prohibit hiatal hernia reduction. The fundus is vertically divided, and the medial portion is used to lengthen the distal esophagus into a 3–6 cm conduit, which is surrounded by a 360° fundal wrap.

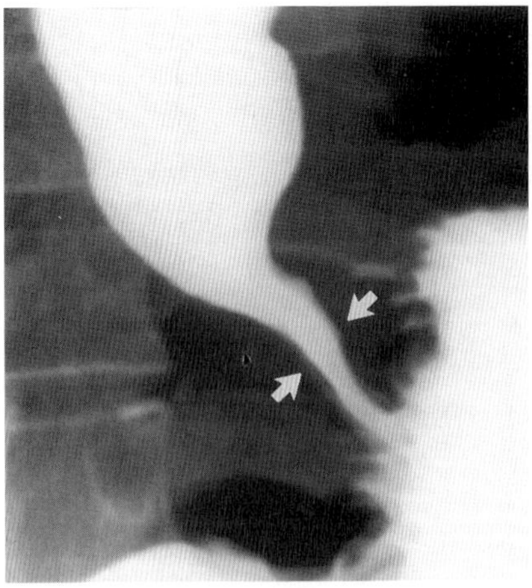

FIGURE 1. *Gastric fundoplication anatomy. The gastric fundus is wrapped around the distal esophagus (arrows).*

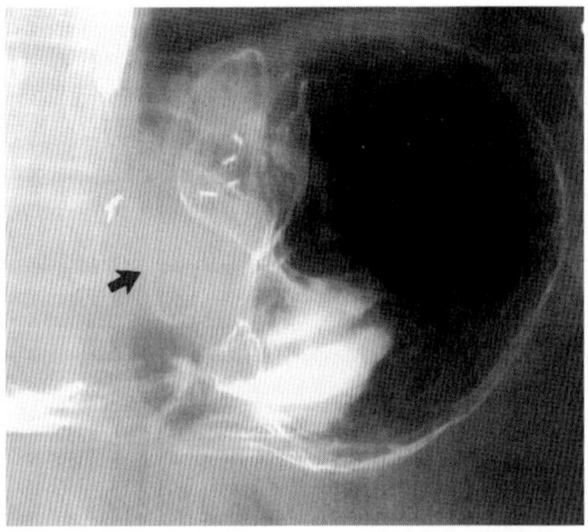

FIGURE 2. *Angelchik antireflux prosthesis. A freely movable silicone prosthesis is placed around the distal esophagus, between the diaphragm and the stomach. A tantalum band (arrow) serves as the radiographic marker.*

EXAM

1 *Obtain Clinical History*

Knowledge of the patient's type of fundoplication is essential. For hiatal hernia repair, the basic operation involves reducing the hernia and wrapping the fundus around the abdominal esophagus. There are multiple variations employing different degrees of circumferential wrap. They all produce a pseudotumor defect. Contact the referring clinician for a description of the type of surgery performed and to learn the reason for performing the exam.

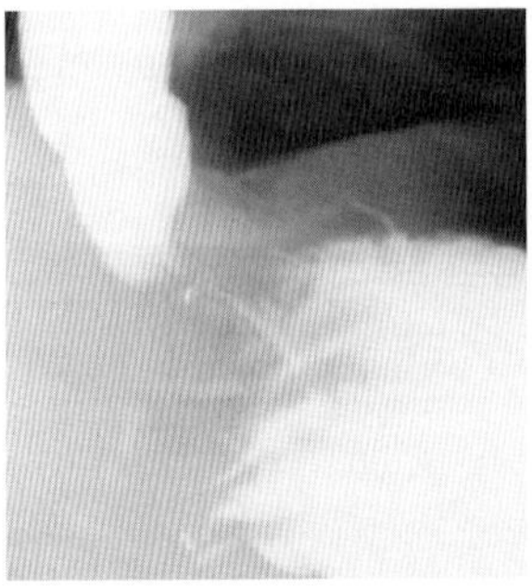

10 × 12
1 on 1
or
spot film

2 *Image Gastroesophageal Junction*

If the purpose is to rule out a postoperative leak, begin the procedure with water-soluble contrast. If no leak is visualized, continue with regular barium.

Have the patient drink 6–8 oz contrast and begin imaging as it reaches the distal esophagus, which is usually narrowed as it passes through the wrap.

TABLETOP
Horizontal

110 kVp

PATIENT
LPO

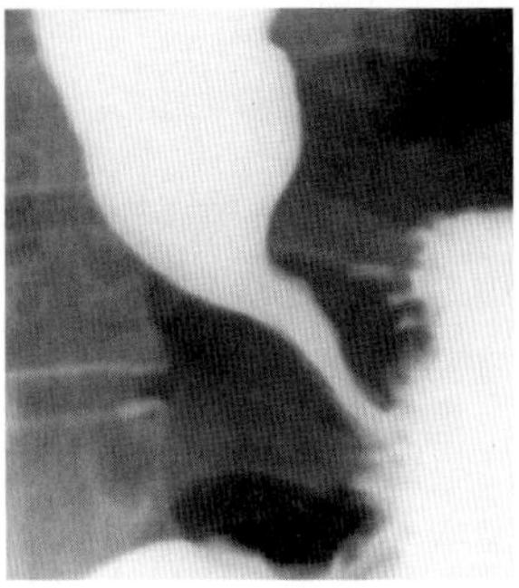

10 × 12
1 on 1
or
spot film

3 *Image Proximal Stomach*

Image the proximal stomach in different obliquities as the patient is turned from left to right. Obtain additional images when the pseudotumor defect is seen.

TABLETOP
Horizontal

PATIENT
LPO → RPO

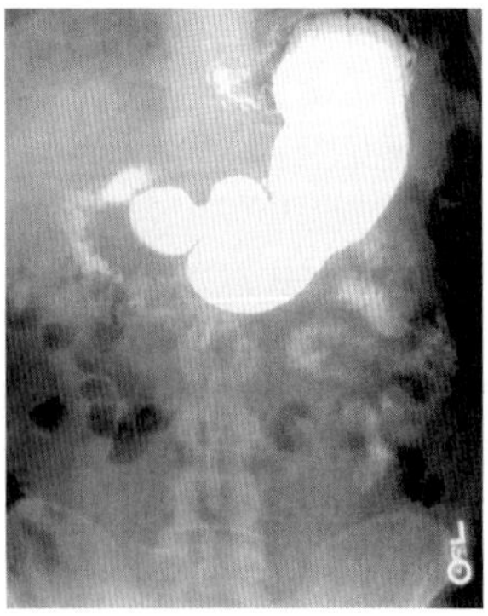

14 × 17

4 *Obtain Overhead Film*

Have the technologist obtain an overhead film of the abdomen. ■

TABLETOP
Horizontal

90 kVp

PATIENT
AP/PA

Vertical Gastric Banding Evaluation

INDICATIONS

- Vertical gastric banding

CONTRAINDICATIONS

- Postoperative exams to exclude leakage should be performed with water-soluble contrast

PATIENT PREPARATION

- NPO after midnight or 6 hours prior to exam

SUPPLIES

- 6 oz regular barium (60% w/v)
- ±4–8 oz chilled 37% iodine water-soluble gastrointestinal contrast (e.g., Gastrografin, MD-Gastroview)
- Barium cup
- Large-caliber flexible straw

SCOUT FILM

- AP abdomen

SAMPLE DICTATION

A limited upper gastrointestinal series was performed to evaluate the patient's recent vertical gastric banding. As the procedure was ordered to exclude a postoperative leak, Gastrografin was initially used, followed with regular barium. Contrast initially accumulated in the gastric pouch, then slowly drained through a narrow channel into the remainder of the stomach. No postoperative leakage of contrast was identified. The visualized portions of the proximal small bowel are unremarkable. ■

RADIATION

- Fluoro: 650 mrad/min
- Spot films: 50 rad per spot film

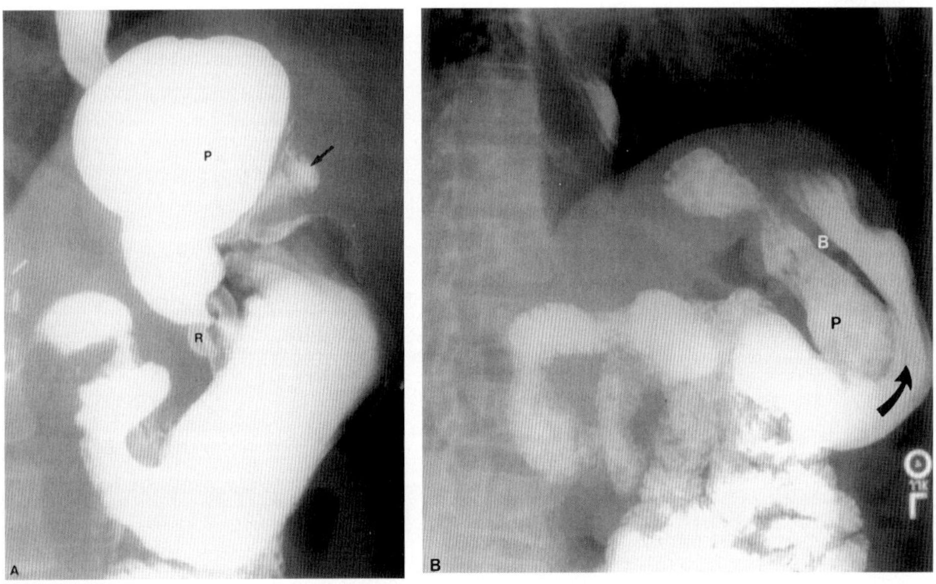

B—vertical gastric band (staple line)
P—pouch
R—silicone ring
arrow—contrast refluxed into proximal stomach on other side of band

FIGURE 1. *Postoperative anatomic variants of vertical gastric banding.*

EXAM

1 Obtain Clinical History

Contact the referring clinician for a description of the type of surgery performed and to learn the reason for performing the exam.

If the purpose is to rule out a postoperative leak, begin the procedure with water-soluble contrast. If no leak is visualized, continue with regular barium.

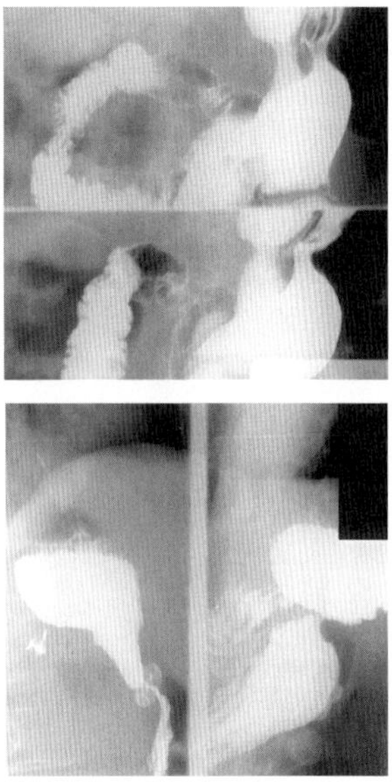

10 × 12
2 on 1
or
spot film

2 Image Pouch

Locate the suture lines on the scout film. Have the patient drink 4 oz contrast and search for the staple line by turning the patient from left to right, imaging as you do this.

The vertical gastric band will appear as a vertical dark line outlined by the contrast. The contrast should initially be contained in the pouch medial to the band, and then begin to empty through a "ring" at the bottom of the pouch.

TABLETOP
Head Up
45°

110 kVp

PATIENT
LPO → RPO

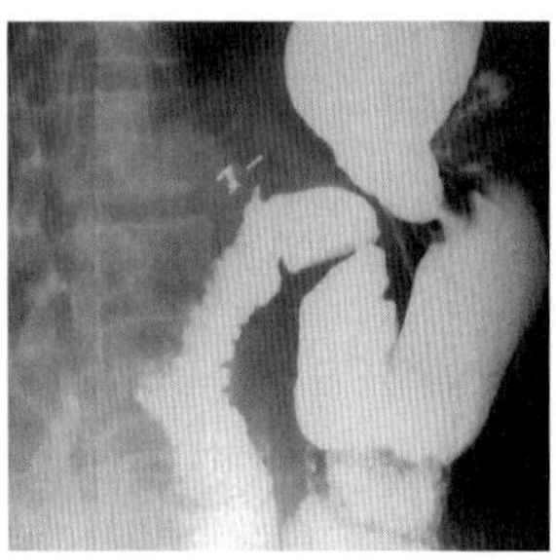

10 × 12
1 on 1
or
spot film

3 Image Distal Stomach

Keep the patient in the head-up position to promote further filling of distal stomach and duodenum.

TABLETOP
Head Up
45°

PATIENT
AP

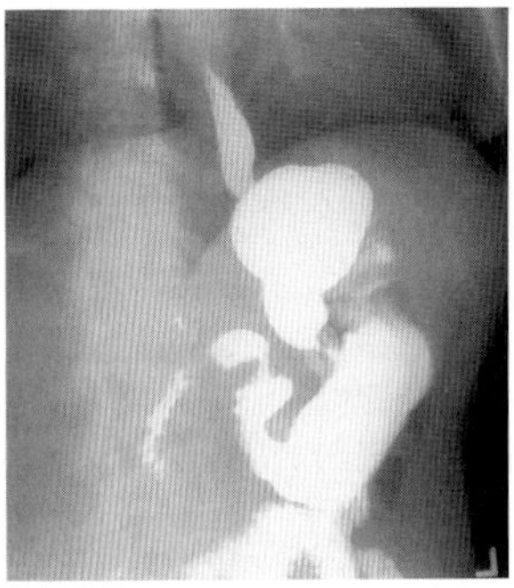

14 × 14
1 on 1

4 *Image Entire Stomach*

Using a single 14 × 14 film, image the entire stomach.

A small amount of contrast may reflux from the distal stomach along the lateral side of the band, making it visible.

TABLETOP

Horizontal

PATIENT

AP

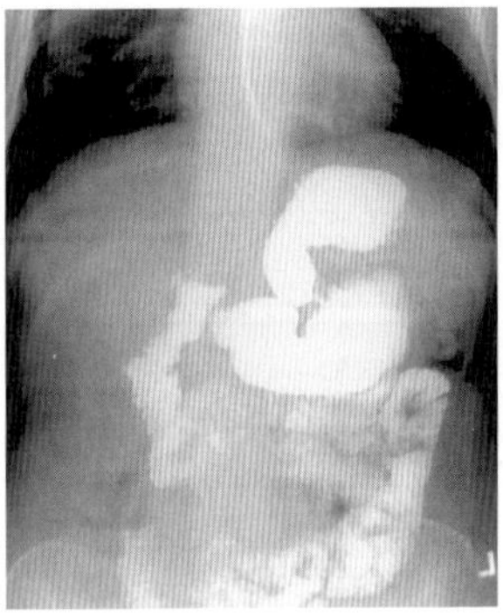

14 × 17

5 *Obtain Overhead Film*

Obtain an overhead AP film. ■

TABLETOP

Horizontal

90 kVp

PATIENT

AP

Billroth Evaluation

INDICATIONS

- Billroth I (partial gastrectomy with gastroduodenal anastomosis)
- Billroth II (partial gastrectomy with gastrojejunal anastomosis)

CONTRAINDICATIONS

- Postoperative exams to exclude leakage should be performed with water-soluble contrast

PATIENT PREPARATION

- NPO after midnight or 6 hours prior to exam

SUPPLIES

- 4–6 oz dense barium (200–250% w/v)
- Barium cup
- 3/4 ampule effervescent granules (e.g., Baros)
- 10 cc water
- 2 medicine cups (for effervescent granules and water)

SCOUT FILM

- AP abdomen

SAMPLE DICTATION

A double contrast upper gastrointestinal series was performed to evaluate the patient's Billroth I gastroduodenostomy. The esophagus and gastric remnant have a normal appearance. The gastroduodenal anastomosis has a normal appearance. There is no evidence of stricture or recurrent tumor. The visualized portions of the proximal small bowel are unremarkable. ■

RADIATION

- Fluoro: 650 mrad/min
- Spot films: 50 mrad per spot film

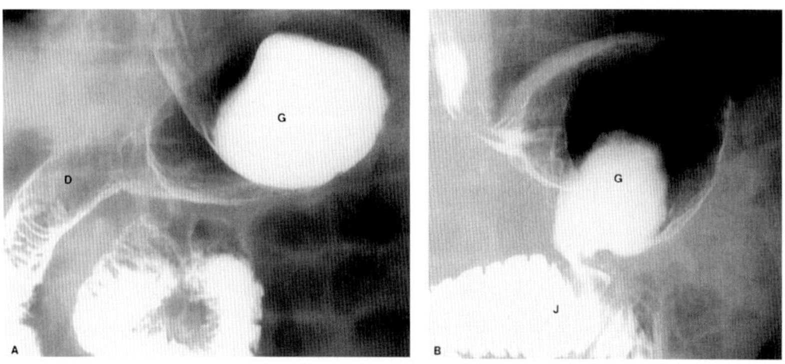

G—gastric remnant
D—duodenal remnant
J—jejunum

FIGURE 1. *Postoperative Billroth I (A) and Billroth II (B) anatomy.*

EXAM

1 Obtain Clinical History

Contact the referring clinician for a description of the type of surgery performed and to learn the reason for performing the exam.

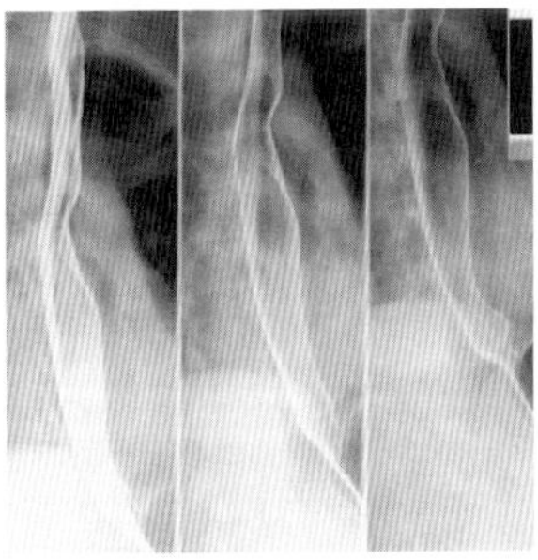

2 Scan Esophagus

With the tabletop elevated to 45°, place the effervescent granules and 10 cc water in the patient's mouth. Have the patient swallow and then quickly drink 4 oz dense barium. Caution the patient not to burp.

Scan the esophagus and as the stomach begins to fill, move the tabletop to the horizontal position to prevent too much spillage from the anastomosis.

TABLETOP
Head Up
45°

90 kVp

PATIENT
AP

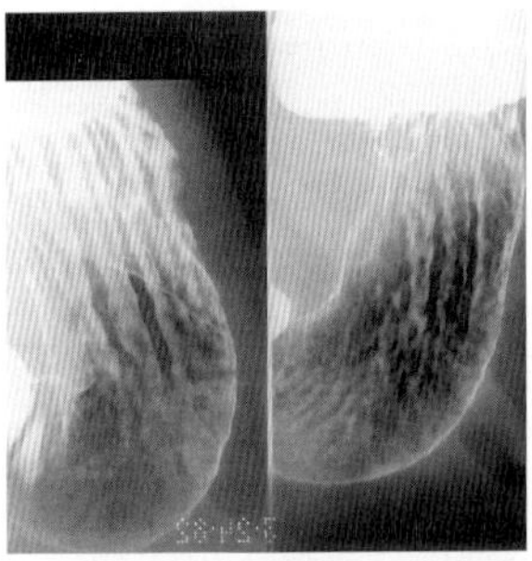

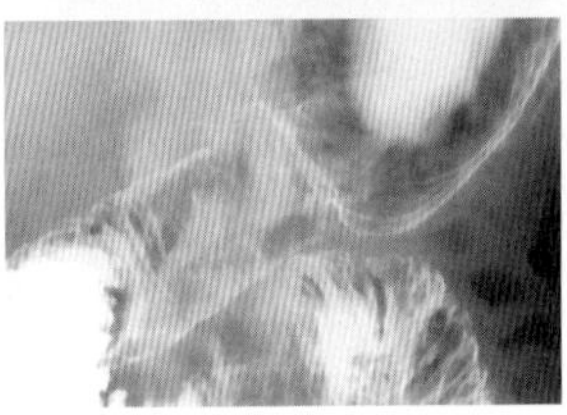

10 × 12
1–2 on 1
or
spot films

3 Image Stomach

Immediately place the patient prone, then rock the hips to and fro 8–10 times to optimize mucosal coating. Image the stomach in the following projections:

1. AP
2. RPO
3. LPO

TABLETOP
Horizontal

PATIENT
AP
RPO
LPO

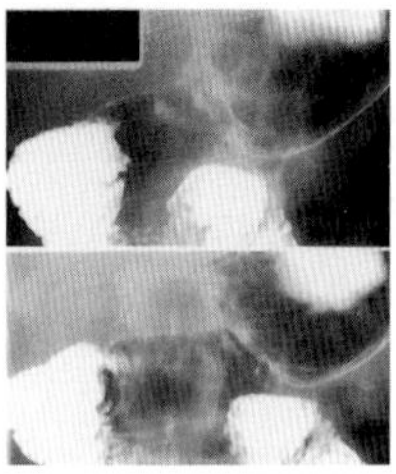

10 × 12
2–4 on 1
or
spot films

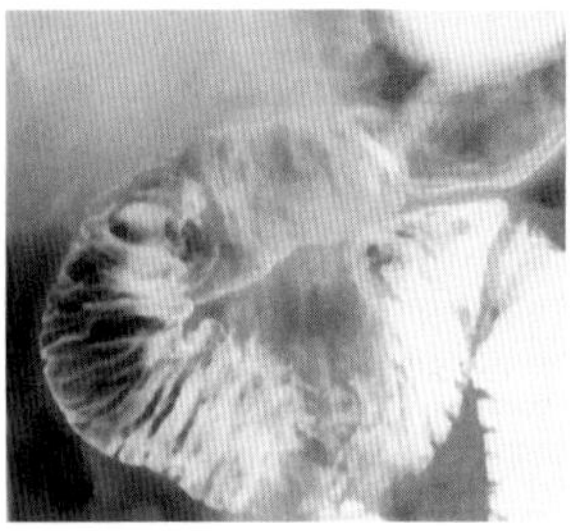

1 on 1
or
spot film

4a *Image Gastroduodenal Anastomosis (Billroth I)*

Image the gastroduodenal anastomosis and the remainder of the duodenum.

TABLETOP

Horizontal

PATIENT

AP

Various obliques

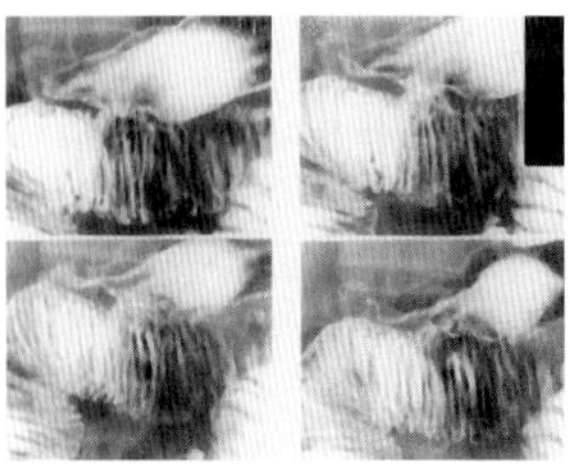

10 × 12
2–4 on 1
or
spot films

4b *Image Gastrojejunal Anastomosis (Billroth II)*

Image the gastrojejunal anastomosis.

TABLETOP

Horizontal

PATIENT

AP

Various obliques

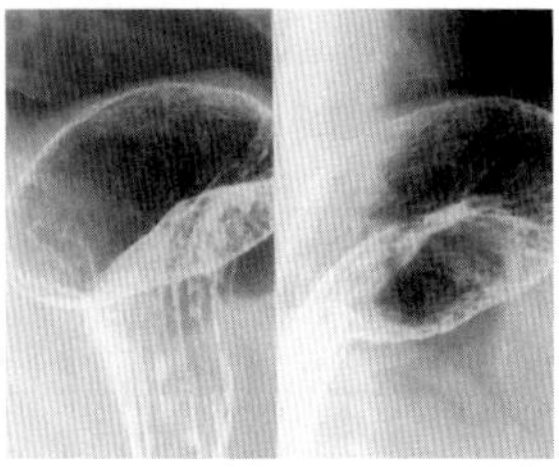

10 × 12
2 on 1
or
spot film

5 *Image Gastric Fundus*

Turn the patient to the right lateral position and film the fundus, or bring tabletop to the vertical position and film the fundus in AP and LPO projections.

It may be necessary to have the patient retract overlying breast tissue to avoid unnecessary irradiation and image degradation.

TABLETOP

Horizontal

±Vertical

PATIENT

Rt Lat

±AP/LPO

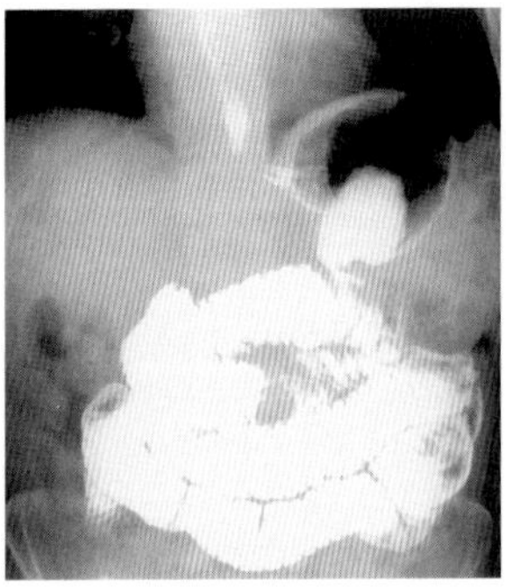

14 × 17

6 *Obtain Overhead Film*

Have the technologist obtain an overhead PA film. ■

TABLETOP
Horizontal

90 kVp

PATIENT
PA

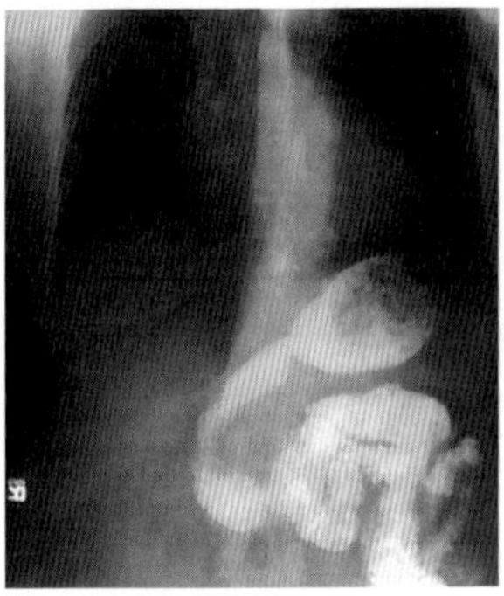

14 × 17

✪ *Single Contrast Billroth Upper Gastrointestinal Series*

Single contrast technique can also be employed for imaging post-Billroth I and II patients by using 6–8 oz regular barium (60% w/v) or chilled 37% iodine water-soluble gastrointestinal contrast (e.g., Gastrografin, MD-Gastroview). Use the same sequence as described above, omitting the effervescent granules. ■

TABLETOP
Horizontal

90 kVp

PATIENT
PA

Enteric Feeding Tube Placement

INDICATIONS

- Inability to place enteric feeding tube correctly without fluoroscopic guidance

CONTRAINDICATIONS

- Nasal route is contraindicated in patients with facial fractures

PATIENT PREPARATION

- NPO after midnight or 6 hours prior to exam

SUPPLIES

- 10 mg (2 cc) metoclopramide
- 3 cc syringe (for metoclopramide)
- 18 gauge needle (for drawing metoclopramide)
- 25 gauge needle (for injecting metoclopramide)
- Tourniquet
- Alcohol
- Small bandage
- Assortment of enteric tubes with guidewires
- 0.0625 inch guidewire
- Silicone spray (for guidewire)
- 2% viscous lidocaine gel
- 3 cc syringe (for lidocaine gel)
- Topical anesthetic spray (e.g., Cetacaine)
- 60 cc catheter tip syringe (for injecting air/contrast)
- ±4–8 oz 37% iodine water-soluble gastrointestinal contrast (e.g., Gastrografin, MD-Gastroview)
- Tincture of benzoin
- 4 × 4 or 2 × 2 gauze (for applying tincture of benzoin)
- Silk tape

SCOUT FILM

- Not obtained routinely

SAMPLE DICTATION

Successful placement of a 12 Fr Entriflex enteric feeding tube into the fourth portion of the duodenum was achieved after 2 minutes of pulsed fluoroscopy. ■

RADIATION

- Fluoro: 650 mrad/min
- Pulsed fluoro: 325 mrad/min
- Spot film: 50 mrad per spot film

EXAM

℞

1 *Administer Metoclopramide*

If not contraindicated, administer 10 mg metoclopramide (intravenously if possible) over 30–60 seconds, as a rapid bolus can result in a feeling of anxiety followed by drowsiness. Metoclopramide relaxes the pylorus and increases antral and small bowel peristalsis to aid in intubation.

TABLETOP

Head Up
30°

PATIENT

AP

℞

2 *Administer Topical Anesthetic*

Lubricate the enteric feeding tube tip with 2% viscous lidocaine gel. The nasopharynx can be anesthetized by injecting additional lidocaine gel with a 3 cc syringe into the nostril and having the patient sniff while occluding the contralateral nostril.

If an oral approach is to be used, the oropharynx can be anesthetized with topical spray.

TABLETOP
Horizontal

PATIENT
AP/Sitting

3 *Prepare Tube*

Read the instructions that are packaged with the enteric feeding tube. Some tubes require flushing with water before inserting the wire stiffener. Other tubes come with the stiffener in place. If a wire stiffener is already loaded into the tube, make sure that it is freely movable before placing it in the patient, as stiffeners can occasionally become tightly adherent to the tube.

If a separate guidewire will be used, it should be lubricated with silicone spray before being inserted into the tube.

TABLETOP
Horizontal

PATIENT
AP/Sitting

4 *Insert Tube into Esophagus*

Insert the tube with wire stiffener in place (but retracted several centimeters to allow flexibility) into the nostril and advance it along the hard palate to the nasopharynx (avoid pushing the tube up into the turbinates). With the patient's neck flexed, continue advancing the tube.

If this results in vigorous coughing, retract the tube slightly and place the patient in the right lateral position to allow visualization of the pharynx. Advance the tube into the esophagus using fluoroscopic visualization.

If the patient does not cough, advance the tube continuously until some resistance is felt; then stop advancing.

TABLETOP
Horizontal

PATIENT
AP/Sitting
±Rt Lat

5 *Advance Tube into Stomach*

Place the patient supine and position the fluoroscope over the stomach. Have the technologist operate the fluoroscope for you or use the foot pedal. Advance the tube into the stomach under fluoroscopic visualization.

It is preferable to use pulsed fluoroscopy for enteric feeding tube placement, as this will decrease the amount of radiation exposure. This procedure can occasionally result in prolonged fluoroscopy time to achieve correct tube placement.

TABLETOP
Horizontal

Pulsed fluoro
7.5 fr/sec
75 kVp

PATIENT
AP

6 *Assess Gastric Distention*

When the tube is in the stomach, observe for the amount of air present. If little or no air is present, withdraw the stylet and inject about 100 cc air using a 60 cc syringe. If the stomach is overly distended with air, withdraw some air using a 60 cc syringe. Replace the wire stiffener under fluoroscopic visualization. Never advance a wire stiffener without fluoroscopic guidance, as the wire tip can exit through a side port of the tube and result in visceral perforation.

TABLETOP
Horizontal

PATIENT
AP

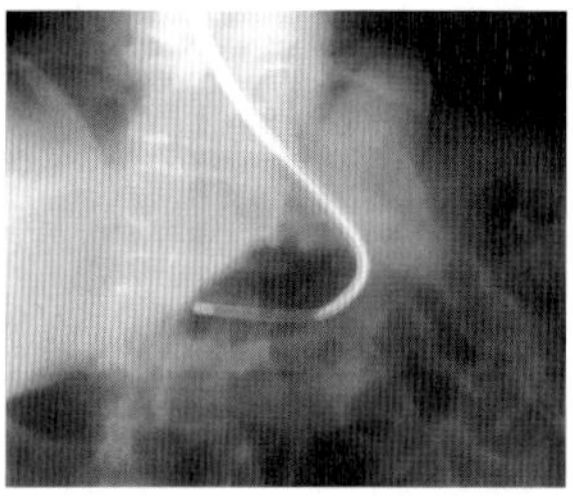

7a *Tip Near Pylorus*

If the tip of the tube is pointing toward the pylorus, simply advance the tube. If the tube enters the pylorus and points inferiorly, advance it as far as possible.

If the tube approaches the pylorus, elevates, and points slightly to the right, it is most likely entering the pylorus.

TABLETOP
Horizontal

PATIENT
AP

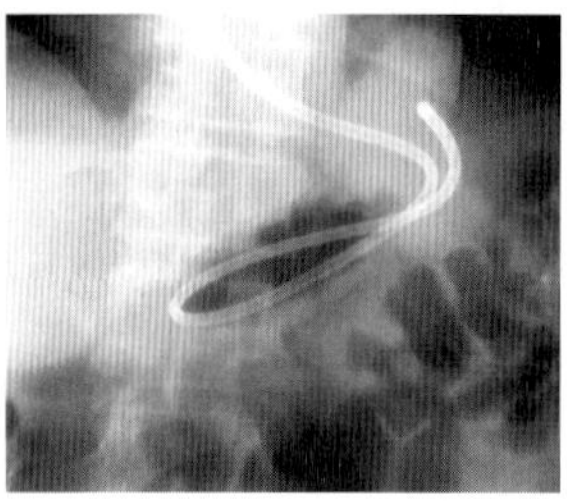

7b *Tube Coiled in Proximal Stomach*

If the tube starts to coil in the proximal stomach, pull the wire stiffener back several centimeters and advance the tube by letting it "double-back" into the middle or distal stomach. Then force the wire stiffener toward the curve of the tube, as this pressure will bring the tip distally. As the tip moves distally, pulling the tube back will aid it in "flipping." Advance the tube into the duodenum.

TABLETOP
Horizontal

PATIENT
AP

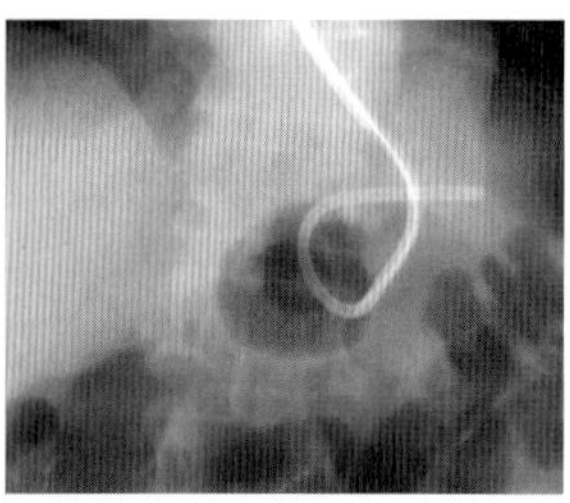

7c *Tube Coiled in Distal Stomach*

If the tube coils in the distal stomach, turn the patient into the left lateral position and try again. If that fails, try to withdraw the cable a few centimeters to allow flexibility and then try again.

TABLETOP
Horizontal

PATIENT
Lt Lat

8 *Alternative Enteric Feeding Tubes*

If continued manipulation of the tube is unsuccessful, try another tube. Common enteric feeding tubes include:

1. Corflo Ultra Lite 8 and 10 Fr 43 inches
2. Entriflex 12 Fr 43 inches
3. Fredrick-Miller 8 Fr 120 cm
4. Ring-McLean 9.5 Fr 130 cm
5. Many other tubes are available

TABLETOP
Horizontal

PATIENT
AP

8 *Alternative Enteric Feeding Tubes* (continued)

If necessary, water-soluble contrast can be injected into the stomach to allow improved visualization of the patient's anatomy.

If the tube cannot be placed in less than 10 minutes of fluoroscopy time, endoscopic placement should be considered to avoid excessive radiation exposure.

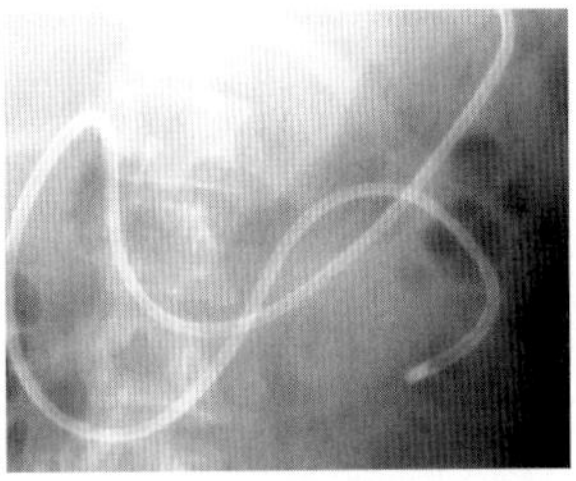

14 × 14
1 on 1

9 *Document Tube Placement*

Document the tube placement with a 14 × 14 film.

TABLETOP
Horizontal

PATIENT
AP

10 *Secure Tube to Patient*

After successful placement, secure the tube to the patient's nose with several pieces of silk tape that are partially bisected longitudinally. Adhesion to the skin can be improved by pretreating the region with a thin coat of tincture of benzoin. ■

TABLETOP
Horizontal

PATIENT
AP

Double Contrast Enteroclysis

INDICATIONS

- Enteroclysis allows detailed visualization of almost every small bowel abnormality (inflammation, infection, neoplasm, adhesions, low-grade small bowel obstruction, mesenteric vascular disease affecting the small bowel, generalized disease, hemorrhage, trauma, aberrant anatomy, etc.)

CONTRAINDICATIONS

- Suspected bowel perforation
- High-grade small bowel obstruction

PATIENT PREPARATION

- NPO after midnight or 6 hours prior to exam

SUPPLIES

- 10 mg (2 cc) metoclopramide
- 3 cc syringe (for metoclopramide)
- 18 gauge needle (for drawing metoclopramide)
- 25 gauge needle (for injecting metoclopramide)
- Tourniquet
- Alcohol swab
- Small bandage
- 12–13 Fr enteroclysis tube (±balloon) with guidewire
- 20 cc syringe (to inflate balloon if a tube with a balloon is used)
- 2% viscous lidocaine gel
- ±Topical anesthetic spray (e.g., Cetacaine)
- 500 cc barium (50–85% w/v)
- 2000 cc 0.5–1.0% w/v methylcellulose solution (e.g., Entrocel, MC)
- 2 barium bags with Y-connector and tubing
- Electric pump
- Silk tape

SCOUT FILM

- AP abdomen

SAMPLE DICTATION

After the intravenous administration of 10 mg metoclopramide, a 12 Fr enteroclysis catheter was placed just beyond the duodenojejunal flexure. Sequential imaging was performed as barium was infused, followed by methylcellulose. The mucosal folds of the jejunum and ileum have a normal appearance throughout. The small bowel is normal in caliber. No strictures, filling defects, or other abnormalities are identified. ■

RADIATION

- Fluoro: 750 mrad/min
- Spot films: 50 mrad per spot film

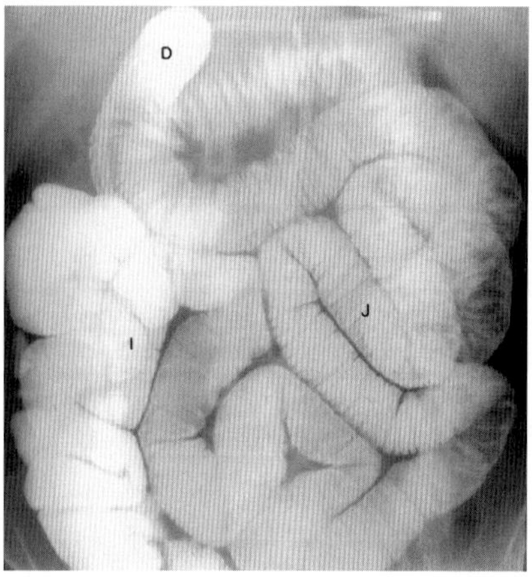

D—duodenum (containing enteroclysis catheter)

J—jejunal loops distended with methylcellulose

I—ileal loops filled with barium

FIGURE 1. *Normal double contrast enteroclysis, using barium followed by methylcellulose.*

EXAM

℞

1 *Administer Metoclopramide*

If not contraindicated, administer 10 mg metoclopramide (intravenously if possible) over 30–60 seconds, as a rapid bolus can result in a feeling of anxiety followed by drowsiness. Metoclopramide relaxes the pylorus and increases antral and small bowel peristalsis to aid in intubation.

TABLETOP
Head Up
20–30°

PATIENT
AP

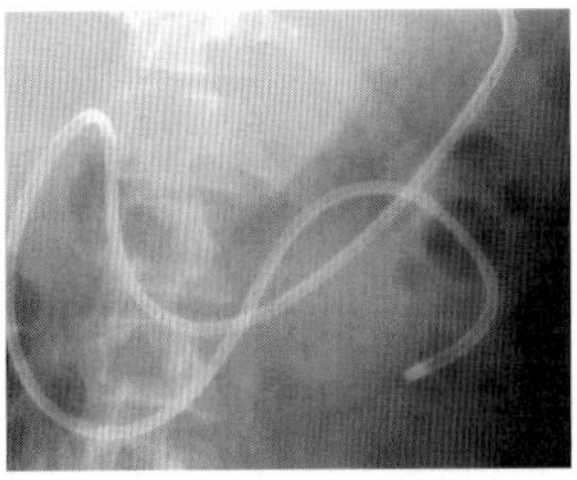

2 *Place Enteroclysis Tube* *(see p. 58)*

Place the enteroclysis tube, using the same technique as for placing an enteric feeding tube. Optimal placement is just beyond the duodenojejunal flexure, but the distal duodenum is also acceptable.

TABLETOP
Horizontal

75 kVp

PATIENT
AP

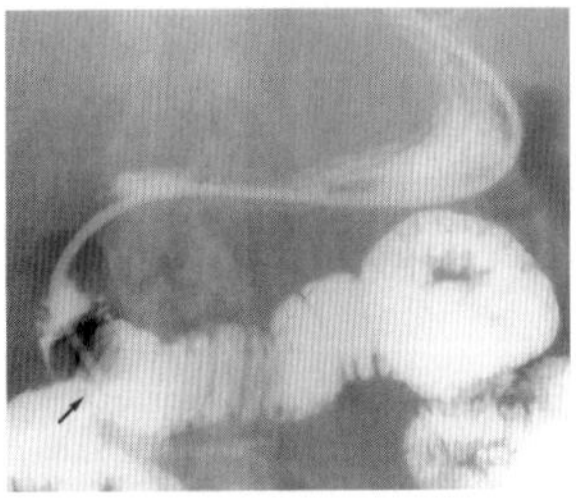

3 *Secure Enteroclysis Tube to Patient*

Secure the tube to the patient's nose with silk tape. If using a tube with a balloon, gently inflate the balloon with up to 15 cc air to secure placement and prevent backflow into the stomach. Tubes with balloons are more expensive but are preferable.

TABLETOP
Horizontal

PATIENT
AP

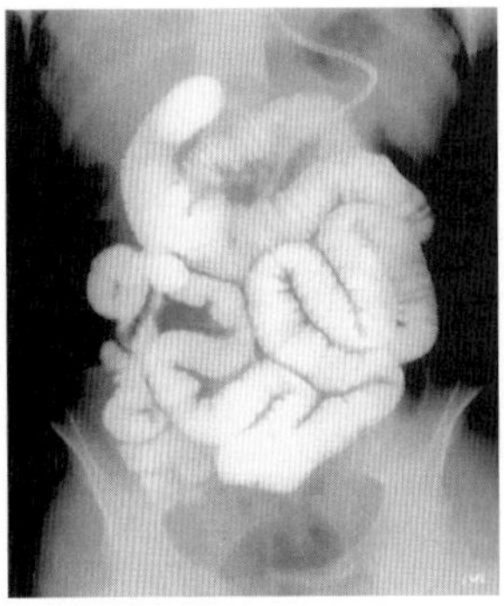

14 × 17
or
14 × 14
1 on 1
or
spot films

4 *Film Proximal Small Bowel*

Begin filling the small bowel with barium at a rate of 125 cc/min. Wait until the jejunal loops are fully distended before filming. Obtain spot films of each group of bowel loops as they are filled with barium, before they become obscured by overlapping subsequently filled loops.

For double contrast technique, stop filling with barium and switch to methylcellulose when the barium-filled loops cross to the right of midline. Obtain spot films of each group of bowel loops as they are filled with methylcellulose.

If an abnormality is identified as filling occurs, obtain spot films in multiple obliquities.

Using a balloon paddle to separate the loops, fluoroscopically inspect all the bowel loops, looking for abnormalities.

TABLETOP
Horizontal

85 kVp

PATIENT
AP

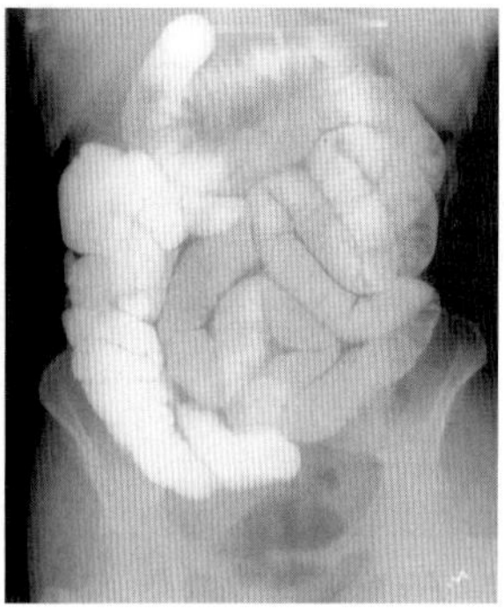

14 × 17
or
14 × 14
1 on 1

5 *Film Distal Small Bowel*

Image the distended ileum as well as the jejunum that is now filled with methylcellulose. Obtain images of the terminal ileum, using spot films if necessary; then stop the pump. It is not necessary to use all of the methycellulose solution.

TABLETOP
Horizontal

PATIENT
AP

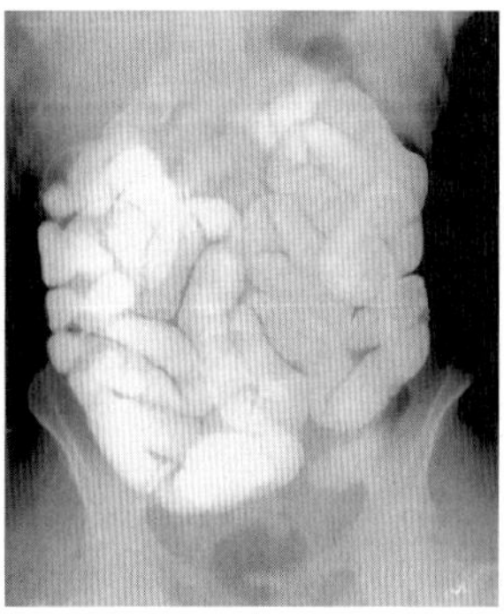

14 × 17

6 *Obtain Overhead Film*

Have the technologist obtain an overhead 85 kVp film.

TABLETOP
Horizontal

85 kVp

PATIENT
AP

7 *Remove Enteroclysis Tube*

Deflate the balloon and remove the enteroclysis tube. ■

TABLETOP
Horizontal

PATIENT
AP

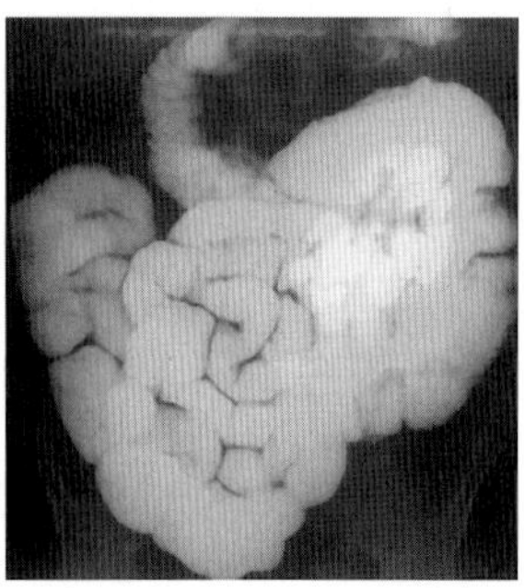

✪ *Single Contrast Enteroclysis*

Single contrast technique can also be used for enteroclysis, particularly for evaluation of small bowel fistulas or obstruction. This examination can be performed using the same technique as for a double contrast examination, except substituting a single bag of 30–40% w/v barium for the two bags of 50–85% barium and methylcellulose.

TABLETOP
Horizontal

90 kVp

PATIENT
AP

✪ ***Single Contrast Enteroclysis*** *(continued)*

In cases of higher-grade small bowel obstruction, it may not be possible to adequately fill the small bowel to the level of the obstruction in an antegrade fashion. Alternatively, the small bowel can be filled retrograde using the same technique as for a single contrast barium enema, using up to 3000 cc of a 12–20% barium suspension. Intravenous administration of 1.0 mg of glucagon and massaging of the ileocecal valve will facilitate retrograde filling of the small bowel. ■

PART III
Colon Examinations

Michael Davis, M.D.
Jeffrey D. Houston, M.D.

Single Contrast Barium Enema

Double Contrast Barium Enema

Salvage Barium Enema

Colostomy Barium Enema

Dynamic Proctography

Colorectal Transit Exam

Single Contrast Barium Enema

INDICATIONS

- Evaluation of masses or polyps ≥1 cm
- Evaluation of strictures
- Bowel obstruction
- Suspected volvulus
- Diverticulitis, diverticulosis
- Screening exams in patients who cannot tolerate a double contrast barium enema
- Advanced infection/inflammation

CONTRAINDICATIONS

- Toxic megacolon
- If bowel perforation is suspected, water-soluble contrast is used by convention.

PATIENT PREPARATION

- On the day prior to the exam, the patient consumes two cartons of a liquid nutritional supplement (e.g., Resource, Ensure) for each breakfast, lunch, and dinner. This provides calories without residue.
- At 2:00 P.M. on the day prior to the exam, the patient drinks 12 oz of magnesium citrate, then drinks 8 oz of water every hour until 6:00 P.M., when four 5 mg bisacodyl laxative tablets are taken.
- The patient then drinks 8 oz water at 7:00 P.M., 8:00 P.M., and 9:00 P.M. on the day prior to the exam.
- A 10 mg bisacodyl suppository is unwrapped and inserted into the rectum between 6:00 A.M. and 7:00 A.M. on the morning of the exam.

SUPPLIES

- ±1.0 mg glucagon
- 1 cc syringe (for glucagon)
- 18 gauge needle (for drawing glucagon)
- 25 gauge needle (for injecting glucagon)
- Tourniquet
- Alcohol swab
- Small bandage
- 500 cc barium (85–100% w/v) mixed into 1500 cc tepid water (to produce a 12–20% w/v solution)
- Barium enema bag and tubing
- Single contrast enema tip with retention cuff
- Lubrication jelly
- Cuff inflator (for enema tip retention cuff)
- ±Inflatable enema ring (if patient appears unable to retain contrast)

SCOUT FILM

- AP

SAMPLE DICTATION

The entire colon was filled with barium. No polyps, diverticula, strictures, masses, or other abnormalities were seen. The terminal ileum is normal in appearance. ■

RADIATION

- Fluoro: 750 mrad/min
- Spot films: 70 mrad per spot film

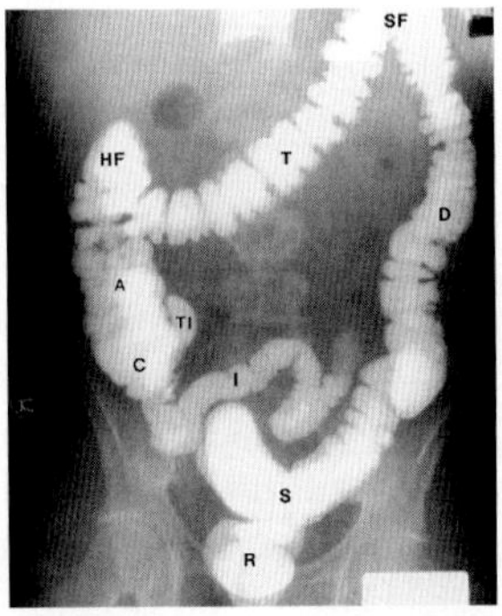

I—ileum
TI—terminal ileum
C—cecum
A—ascending colon
HF—hepatic flexure
T—transverse colon
SF—splenic flexure
D—descending colon
S—sigmoid colon
R—rectum

FIGURE 1. *Normal colonic anatomy.*

EXAM

1 *Inspect Scout Film for Bowel Preparation*

If sufficient retained stool is visualized on the scout film, consider rescheduling the patient for the following day and repeating the bowel preparation or performing a cleansing enema. Residual stool can obscure small colonic lesions.

℞

2 *Administer Glucagon*

Patients ≥60 years: If not contraindicated, administer 1.0 mg glucagon (intravenously if possible). Administer the glucagon slowly, as nausea and other side effects can result from rapid administration.

Patients <60 years: Use glucagon only as needed, usually for spasm.

TABLETOP
Head Up
20–30°

PATIENT
AP

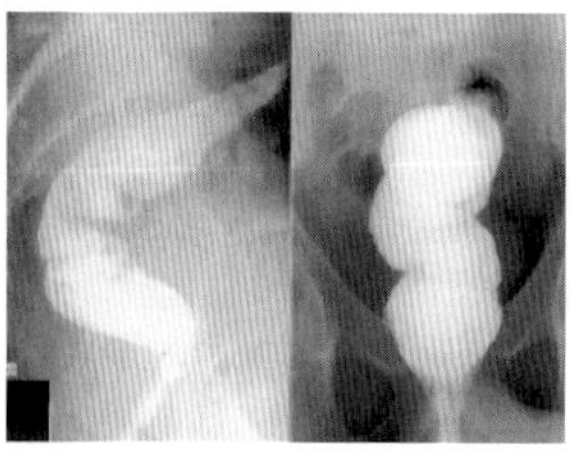

10 × 12
2 on 1
or
spot film

3 *Image Rectum*

With the patient in the Sims position, have the technologist carefully place a lubricated single contrast enema tip into the rectum. Gently inflate a rectal balloon if necessary, observing with fluoroscopy to ensure placement proximal to the internal sphincter.

Fill the rectum until it is distended; then image the rectum in the following projections:

1. Lt Lat
2. AP

TABLETOP
Head Up
20–30°

110 kVp

PATIENT
Lt Lat
AP

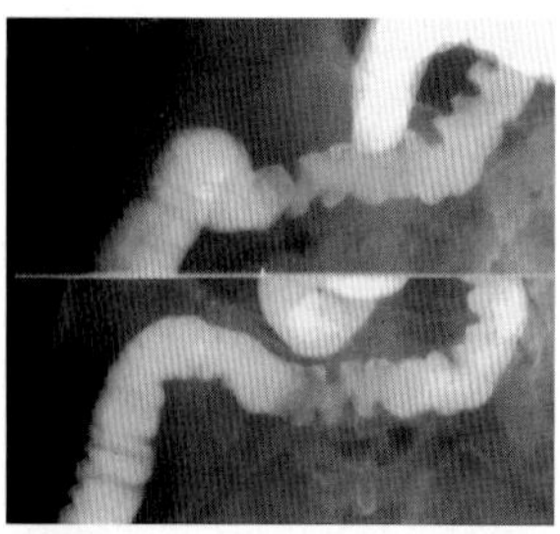

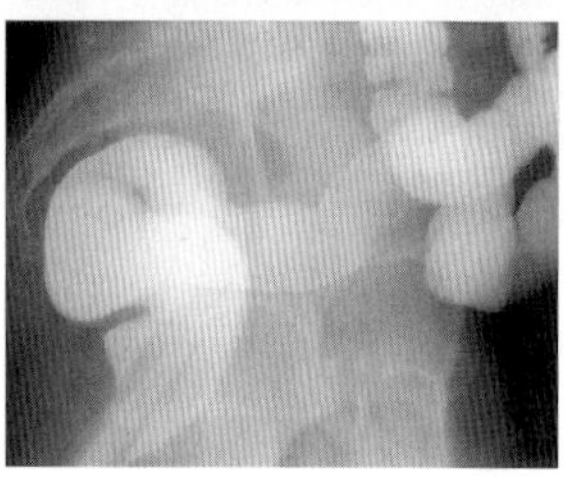

10 × 12
1–2 on 1
or
spot film

4 *Image Sigmoid Colon*

Fill the sigmoid colon. Obtain one or two slightly different views at each position:

1. Sigmoid (LPO)
2. Reverse sigmoid (RPO/Rt Lat)

When filling the colon, remember that if a particular segment seems not to fill adequately, find the head of the barium column. If it is some distance from the segment you are imaging, it will probably not fill any further. Continued filling risks barium flooding the entire colon, terminal ileum, and additional small bowel, and possibly obscuring the rectosigmoid.

TABLETOP
Head Up
20–30°

PATIENT
LPO
RPO/Rt Lat

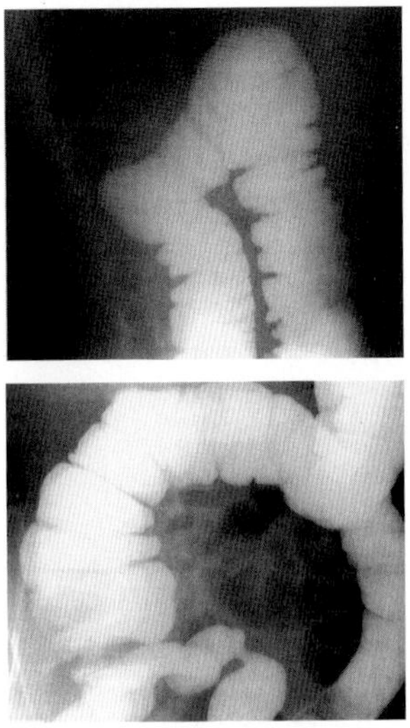

10 × 12
1 on 1
or
spot film

5 *Image Flexures*

Oblique the patient to open and image each flexure:

1. Splenic flexure (RPO)
2. Hepatic flexure (LPO)

TABLETOP
Horizontal

PATIENT
RPO
LPO

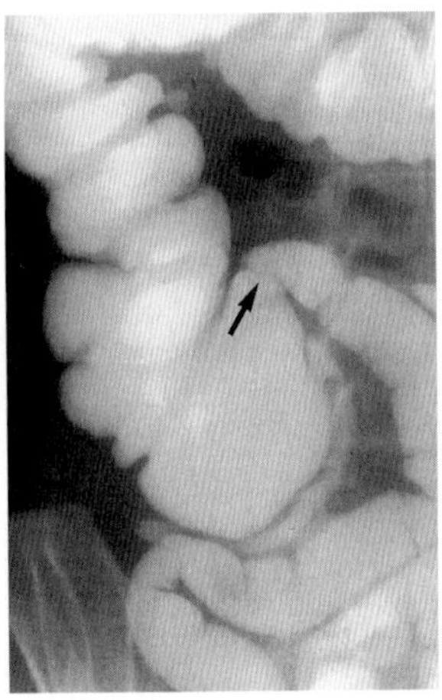

10 × 12
2 on 1
or
spot film
mag

6 *Image Cecum*

Deliver more barium until the cecum is filled. Image with and without compression. The ileocecal valve must be seen to ensure complete filling of the colon.

TABLETOP
Horizontal

PATIENT
AP

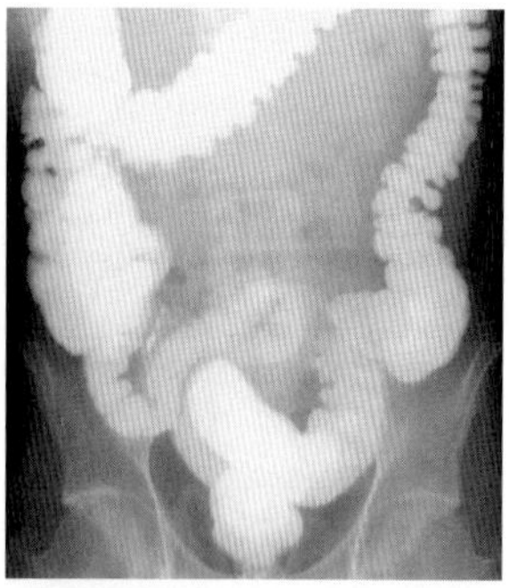

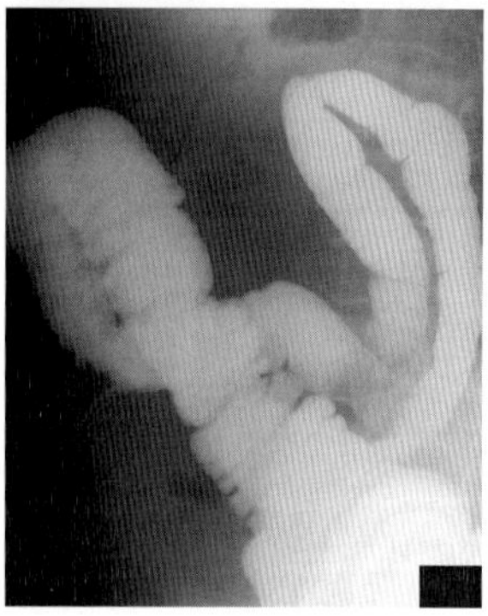

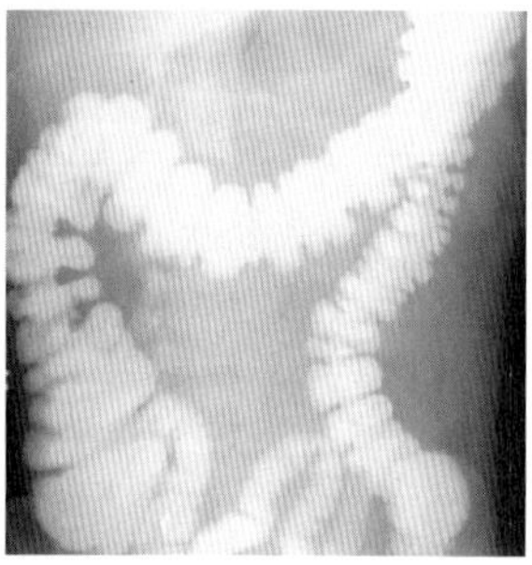

14 × 14
1 on 1

7 Image Entire Colon

Use three 14 × 14 cassettes to image as much of the colon as possible:

1. AP (to include the rectum)
2. RPO (to include both flexures)
3. LPO (to include both flexures)

Remember that the 14 × 14 cassettes have a larger field of view than what is seen on the monitor, so "cut off" some of the image on the monitor, as more will be seen on the film.

TABLETOP
Horizontal

PATIENT
AP
RPO
LPO

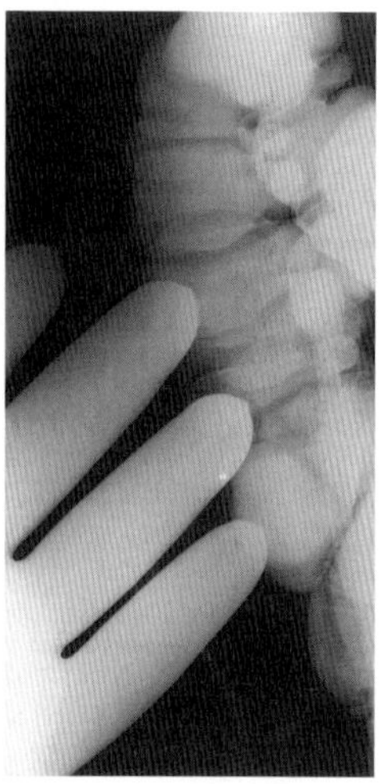

8 Palpate Colon for Masses

Palpate the colon with a lead glove to find masses. Begin with the cecum and work distally. The flexures and rectosigmoid are not palpable.

TABLETOP
Horizontal

PATIENT
AP

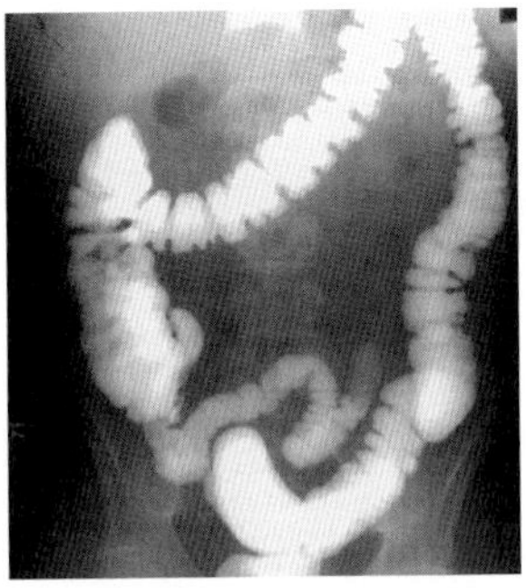

14 × 17

9 ***Obtain Overhead Films***

Have the technologist obtain the following films:

1. AP (to include the rectum)
2. 30° angled sigmoid (AP/LPO)
3. Additional views if needed

TABLETOP

Horizontal

110 kVp

PATIENT

AP/LPO

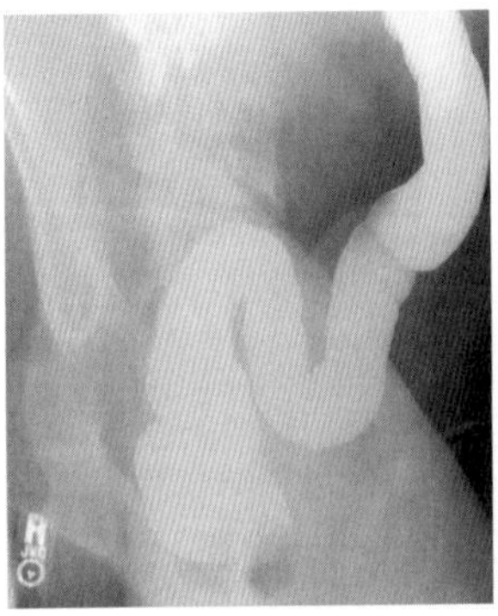

14 × 17

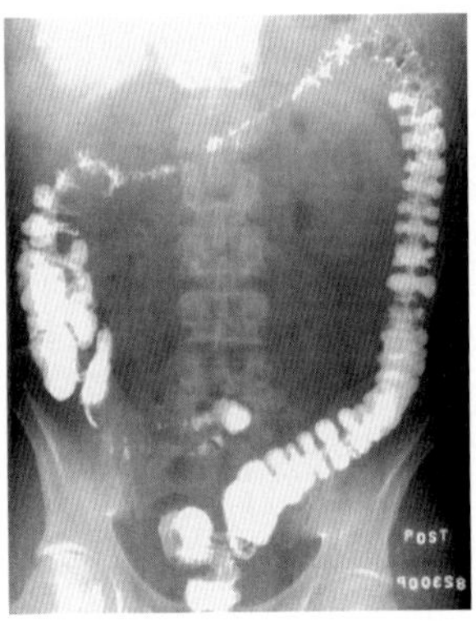

14 × 17

10 ***Obtain Postevacuation Film***

After reviewing the overhead films, send the patient to the restroom to evacuate as much barium as possible, so as to obtain a good postevacuation film. If the patient is having difficulty retaining the barium while on the table, place the enema bag on the floor and unclamp the tube to relieve pressure before sending the patient to the restroom. Have the technologist obtain an overhead AP postevacuation film. ■

TABLETOP

Horizontal

90 kVp

PATIENT

AP

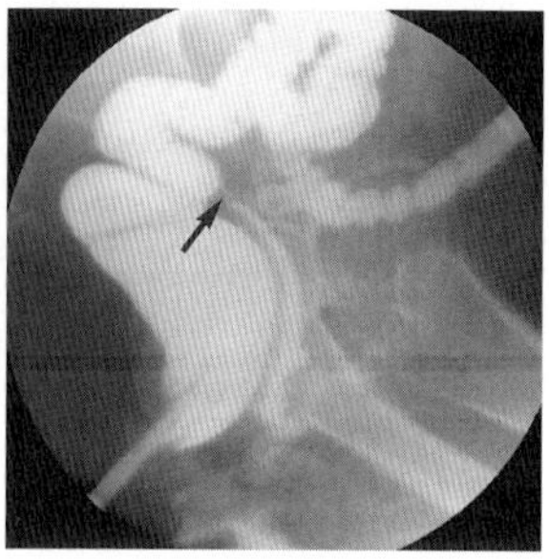

spot film
or
10 × 12
2 on 1

✪ *Rectovaginal Fistula Examination*

Imaging of a rectovaginal fistula can be performed using a single contrast barium enema technique. Place an inflatable enema ring under the patient. Have the technologist carefully insert a single contrast enema tip into the rectum. Do not inflate the rectal balloon. Slowly distend the rectum with barium while closely observing for the fistulous tract. Image the filled tract in multiple obliquities. ■

TABLETOP
Head Up
30°

110 kVp

PATIENT
Lt Lat
Various obliques

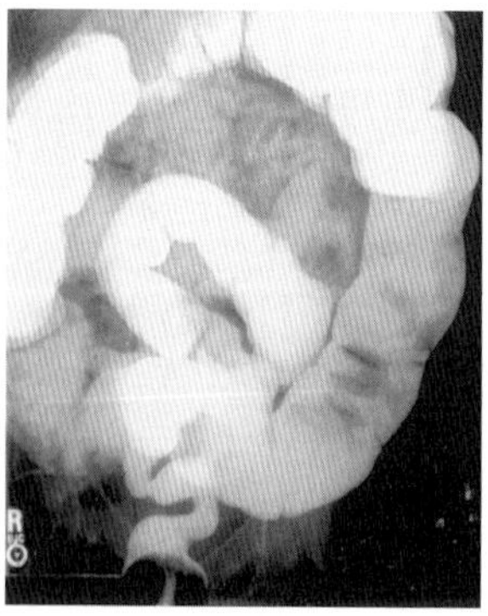

14 × 14
1 on 1

14 × 17

✪ *Therapeutic Water-Soluble Enema*

A therapeutic water-soluble enema can be performed for conditions such as Ogilvie syndrome or fecal impaction.

Do not administer glucagon as it may result in increased paralysis of the bowel. Place an inflatable enema ring under the patient. Have the technologist carefully insert a single contrast enema tip into the rectum. Inflate the retention cuff if necessary, observing with fluoroscopy to ensure placement proximal to the internal sphincter.

Fill the entire colon with up to 2500 cc 14–20% iodine water-soluble contrast (e.g., Cystografin, Cysto-Conray II). Uroradiologic contrast media is routinely used because it is packaged in 500 cc bottles, which conveniently provide the large volume of contrast required for this procedure.

If filling of the right colon is not observed, it may be necessary to place the patient in the right lateral position to facilitate filling.

Obtain two or three 14 × 14 films for documentation. Have the technologist obtain an overhead AP film.

For maximal effect, leave the colon filled for 15 minutes. Alternatively, this examination can be performed in the patient's room using portable radiographs. ■

TABLETOP
Horizontal

75 kVp

PATIENT
AP
LPO
RPO

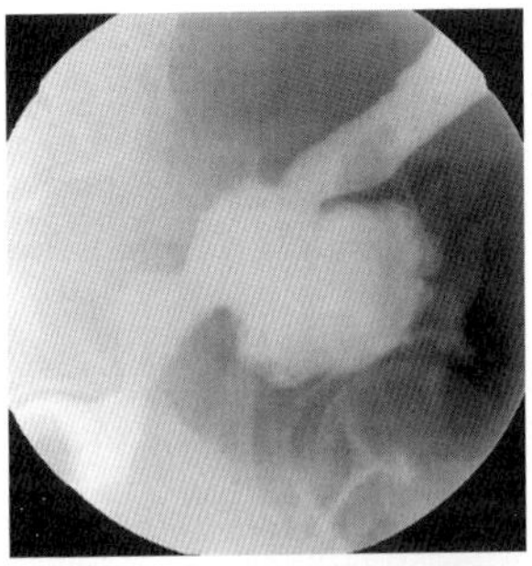

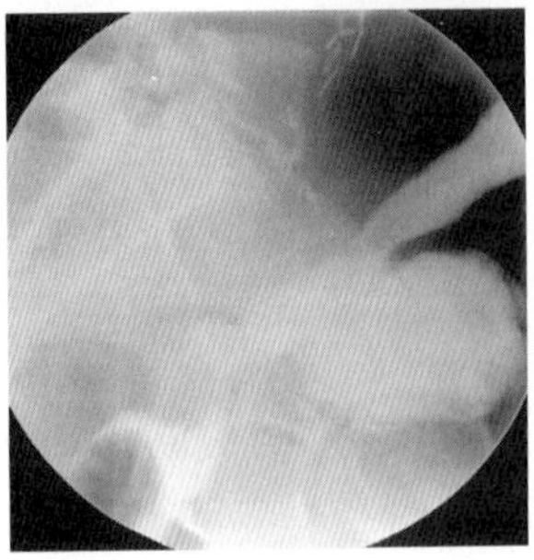

spot film

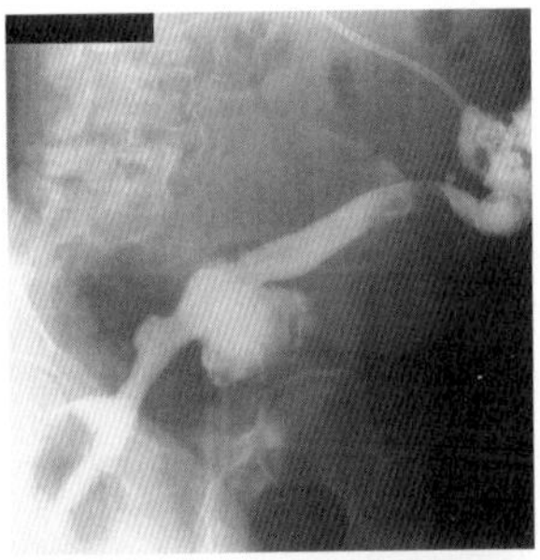

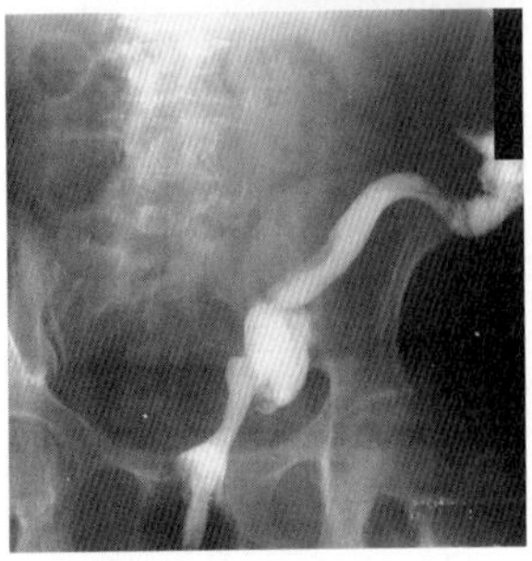

14 × 14
1 on 1

✪ *Water-Soluble Enema to Rule Out Perforation*

If the exam is performed to rule out leakage from a surgical anastomosis, fill just beyond the site of the suspected leak. Take several spot images in different obliquities at the anastomotic site, then several representative 14 × 14 films. ■

TABLETOP

Horizontal

75 kVp

PATIENT

AP

Various obliques

Double Contrast Barium Enema

INDICATIONS

- Routine screening exam for colon carcinoma and polyps <1 cm
- Early infection/inflammation or other mucosal diseases

CONTRAINDICATIONS

- Toxic megacolon
- Suspected bowel perforation
- History of spastic colon (perform single contrast barium enema)
- Poor rectal tone (perform single contrast barium enema)
- Diverticulitis (perform single contrast barium enema to allow filling of intramural sinus tracts)

PATIENT PREPARATION

- On the day prior to the exam, the patient consumes two cartons of a liquid nutritional supplement (e.g., Resource, Ensure) for each breakfast, lunch, and dinner. This provides calories without residue.
- At 2:00 P.M. on the day prior to the exam, the patient drinks 12 oz magnesium citrate, then drinks 8 oz water every hour until 6:00 P.M., when four 5 mg bisacodyl laxative tablets are taken.
- The patient then drinks 8 oz water at 7:00 P.M., 8:00 P.M., and 9:00 P.M. on the day prior to the exam.
- A 10 mg bisacodyl suppository is unwrapped and inserted into the rectum between 6:00 A.M. and 7:00 A.M. on the morning of the exam.

SUPPLIES

- 1.0 mg glucagon
- 1 cc syringe (for glucagon)
- 18 gauge needle (for drawing glucagon)
- 25 gauge needle (for injecting glucagon)
- Tourniquet
- Alcohol swab
- Small bandage
- 500–600 cc barium (105% w/v)
- Barium enema bag with wide tubing (to allow flow of dense barium)
- Double contrast enema tip with retention cuff
- Cuff inflator (for enema tip retention cuff)
- Lubrication jelly
- Pneumatic bulb (to inflate colon)

SCOUT FILM

- AP abdomen

SAMPLE DICTATION

After intravenous administration of 1.0 mg of glucagon, a double contrast barium enema was performed. The entire colon was coated with barium and adequately distended with air. All colonic segments are well visualized and are normal in appearance. ■

RADIATION

- Fluoro: 750 mrad/min
- Spot films: 70 mrad per spot film

EXAM

1 *Inspect Scout Film for Bowel Preparation*

If sufficient retained stool is visualized on the scout film, consider rescheduling the patient for the following day and repeating the bowel preparation or performing a cleansing enema. Residual stool can obscure small colonic lesions.

TABLETOP

Horizontal

PATIENT

AP

℞

2 *Administer Glucagon*

If not contraindicated, administer 1.0 mg glucagon (intravenously if possible). Administer the glucagon slowly, as nausea and other side effects can result from rapid administration.

TABLETOP

Head Up

20–30°

PATIENT

AP

3 *Administer Dense Barium*

With the patient in the Sims position, have the technologist carefully insert a lubricated double contrast enema tip into the rectum. Gently inflate the retention cuff if necessary, observing with fluoroscopy to ensure placement proximal to the internal sphincter.

With the patient in the prone position and while monitoring with fluoroscopy, fill the colon with 350 cc undiluted barium (105% w/v). The remainder of the 500 cc barium remains trapped in the wide tubing.

TABLETOP

Head Down

−30°

90 kVp

PATIENT

Sims

PA

4 *Inflate Colon*

Elevate the tabletop to the horizontal position and place the patient in the LPO position. Then begin slowly inflating the colon with air, using a pneumatic bulb. Slowly administer four or five puffs in each position:

1. LPO
2. Lt Lat
3. LAO
4. PA
5. RAO
6. Rt Lat

When barium is obviously well into the right colon, stop inflating, and place the patient prone.

TABLETOP

Horizontal

PATIENT

LPO

Lt Lat

LAO

PA

RAO

Rt Lat

PA

5 *Drain Excess Barium*

Using a latex glove, hold the tubing just below the enema tip and elevate the table to about 80°. Do not let go of the tube. Visualize the barium-filled rectum under fluoroscopy, and have the technologist unclamp the tubing and drain the excess barium from the rectum. Have the technologist reclamp the tubing.

TABLETOP

Head Up 80°

PATIENT

PA

6 *Image Rectosigmoid*

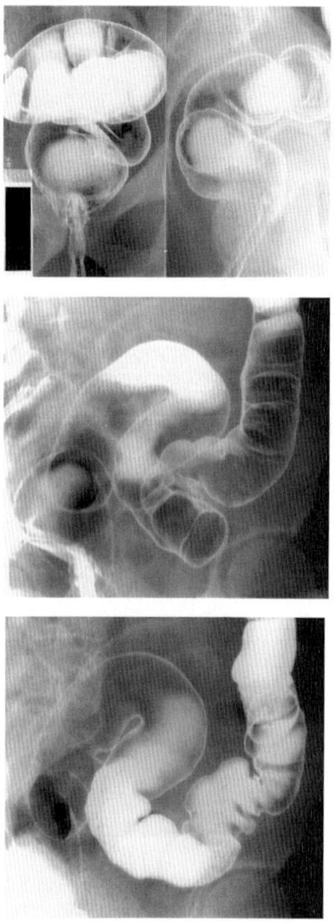

10 × 12
1–2 on 1
or
spot film

Return the table to the horizontal position. Inflate the colon with more air to distend the rectosigmoid; then image the following:

1. Rectum (PA)
2. Rectum (Lt Lat)
3. Sigmoid (LPO)
4. Reverse sigmoid (Rt Lat)

Fully distend the colon with air. Avoid overdistending the colon, which can be uncomfortable for the patient.

TABLETOP

Horizontal

PATIENT

PA

Lt Lat

LPO

Rt Lat

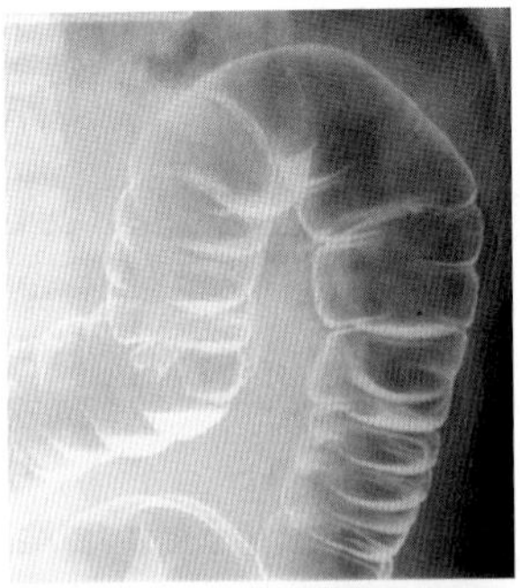

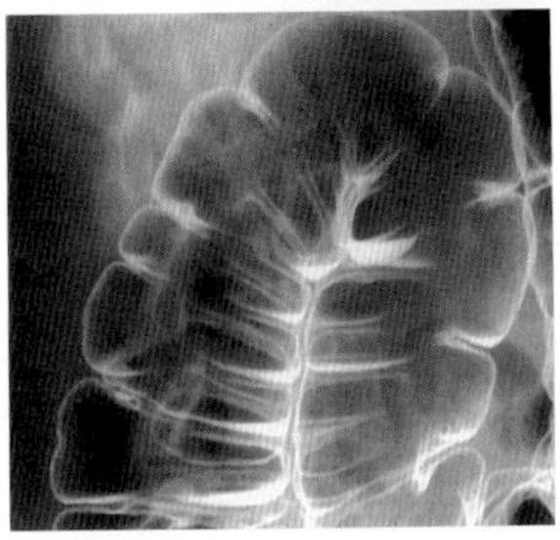

10 × 12
1 on 1
or
spot film

7 Image Flexures

Elevate the table to the upright position. Oblique the patient to open and image each flexure:

1. Splenic flexure (RPO)
2. Hepatic flexure (LPO)

TABLETOP

Vertical

PATIENT

RPO

LPO

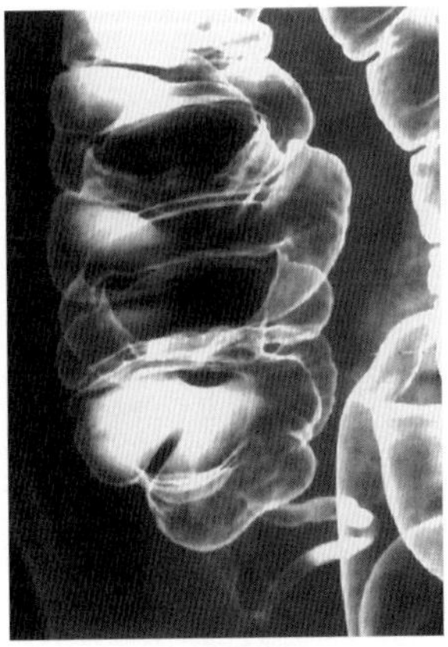

10 × 12
2 on 1
or
spot film

8 Image Cecum

Decline the table to the horizontal position and obtain two slightly different views of the cecum:

1. AP
2. LPO

If barium is retained in the cecum, it may be necessary to decline the tabletop steeply, then turn the patient LPO or RPO and use a lead glove to disperse the barium.

TABLETOP

Horizontal

±Head Down

PATIENT

AP

LPO

±RPO

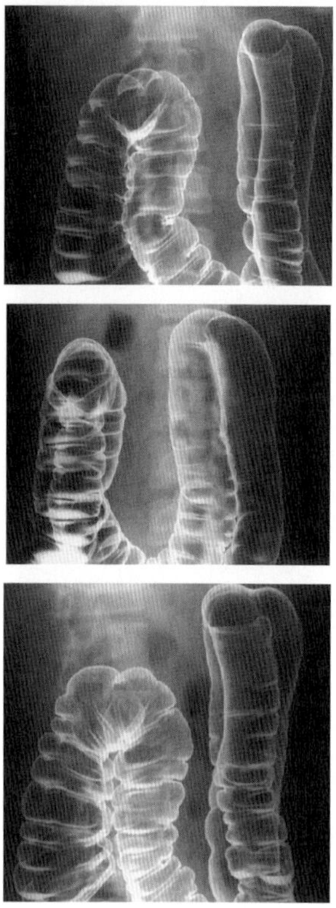

14 × 14
1 on 1

9a *Image Entire Colon*

With 14 × 14 cassettes, obtain the following views of the entire colon:

1. AP (include rectum)
2. RPO (include both flexures)
3. LPO (include both flexures)

TABLETOP

Horizontal

PATIENT

AP

RPO

LPO

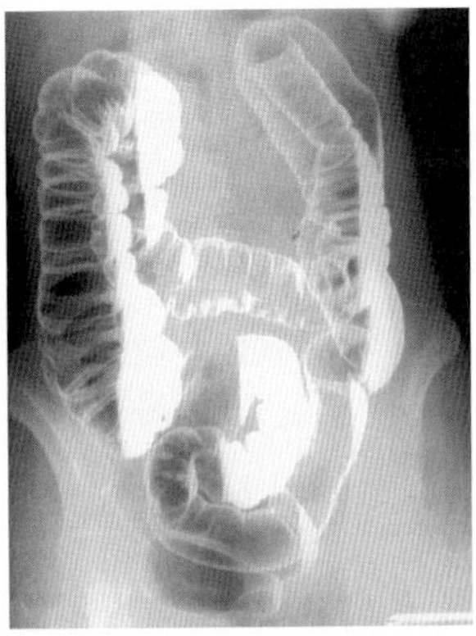

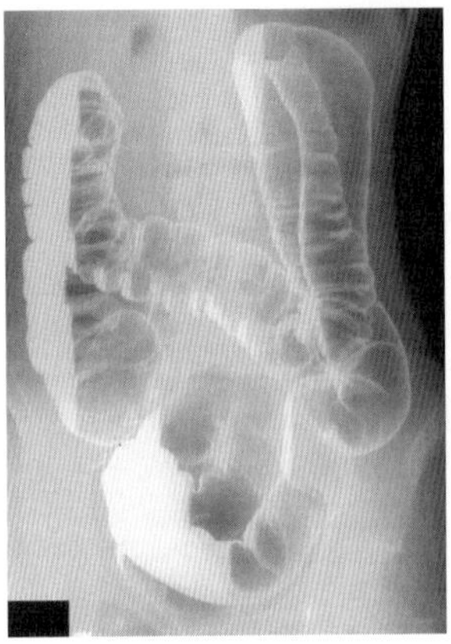

14 × 17

9b ***Image Entire Colon (Alternative)***

Alternatively, imaging of the entire colon can be performed by the technologist:

1. Left lateral decubitus
2. Right lateral decubitus

The edge of the cassette should be positioned at the gluteal crease. This may exclude part of the flexures on some patients, but they have been imaged on spot films.

TABLETOP

Horizontal

PATIENT

Lt Lat

Rt Lat

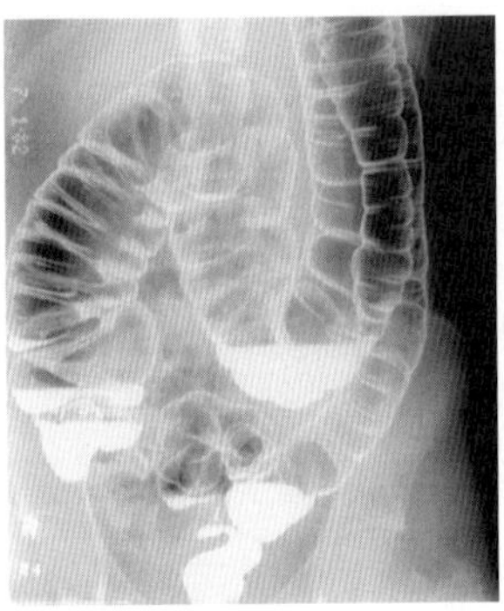

14 × 17

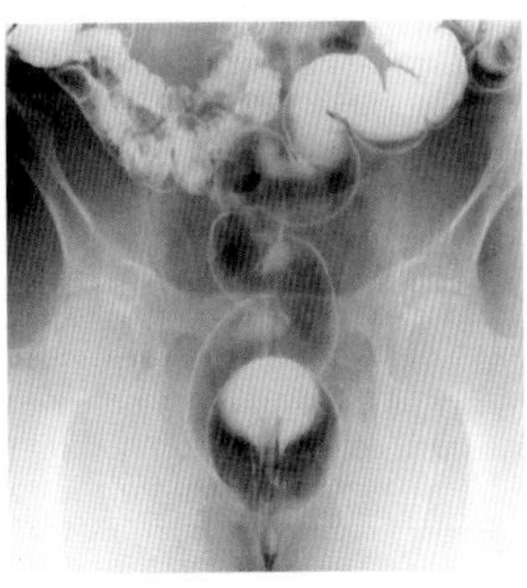

14 × 14

10 ***Obtain Overhead Films***

Have the technologist obtain the following films:

1. AP (to include the rectum; this film can be obtained in the upright position if desired)
2. 30° angled sigmoid (AP/LPO)
3. Additional views if needed

No postevacuation film is needed. ■

TABLETOP

Horizontal
±Vertical

90 kVp

PATIENT

AP/LPO

Salvage Barium Enema

INDICATIONS

- Unsuccessful filling of a colonic segment on double contrast barium enema
- Patient inability to tolerate inflation of the colon on double contrast barium enema

CONTRAINDICATIONS

- See single contrast barium enema

PATIENT PREPARATION

- See double contrast barium enema

SUPPLIES

- 500 cc barium (85–100% w/v) mixed into 1500 cc tepid water (to produce a 12–20% w/v solution)
- Barium enema bag and tubing
- Single contrast enema tip with retention cuff
- Lubrication jelly
- Cuff inflator (for enema tip retention cuff)
- ± Inflatable enema ring (if patient appears unable to retain contrast)

SCOUT FILM

- None

SAMPLE DICTATION

After the intravenous administration of 1.0 mg glucagon, a double contrast barium enema was initially performed. As the double contrast exam was insufficient for visualizing proximal to the hepatic flexure, a salvage barium enema was performed and the right colon was examined by single contrast technique. All colonic segments have a normal appearance. ■

RADIATION

- Fluoro: 1000 mrad/min
- Spot films: 70 mrad per spot film

EXAM

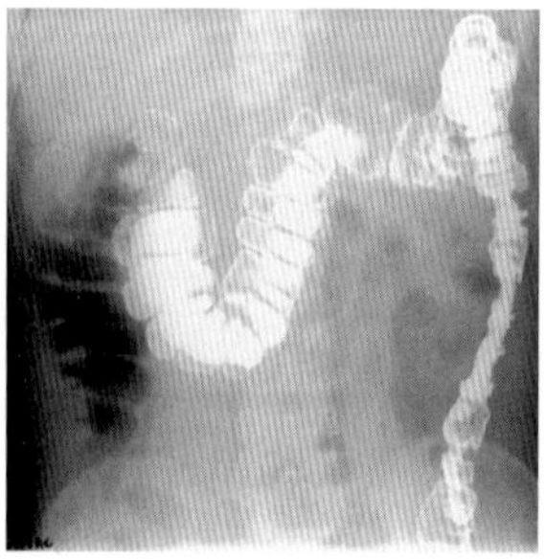

1 ***Perform Double Contrast Barium Enema***

The salvage barium enema is used when part of the colon cannot be examined by the double contrast technique, usually because the colon is too redundant or dense barium cannot be advanced into the ascending colon and cecum.

2 ***Exchange Enema Tip***

When it is apparent that a colonic segment cannot be filled with dense barium, image the segments that are adequately examined by the double contrast technique, including spot films and overhead films. Have the technologist carefully remove the double contrast enema tube and replace it with a single contrast enema tip.

TABLETOP

Horizontal

PATIENT

Sims

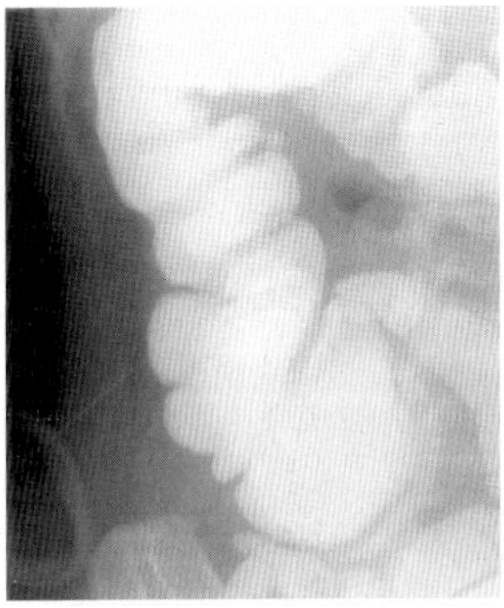

3 *Perform Limited Single Contrast Barium Enema*

Fill the colon as usual for a single contrast barium enema, but image only the previously nonvisualized segments of the colon using spot films and one or two representative overhead films.

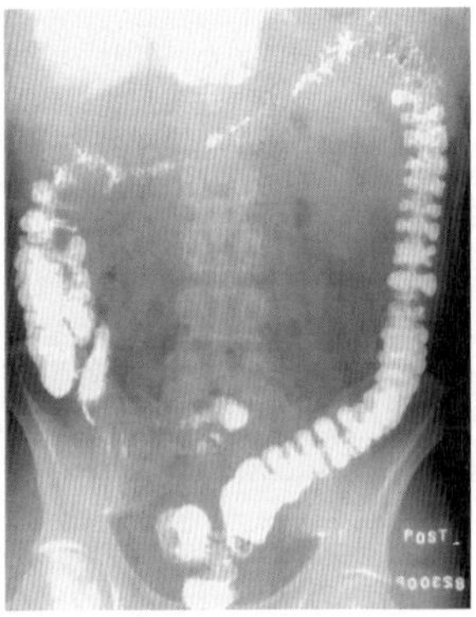

14 × 17

4 *Obtain Postevacuation Film*

Send the patient to the restroom to evacuate as much barium as possible. Have the technologist obtain an overhead AP postevacuation film. ■

TABLETOP

Horizontal

90 kVp

PATIENT

AP

Colostomy Barium Enema

INDICATIONS

- Delineate anatomy in preparation for colostomy revision/takedown

CONTRAINDICATIONS

- Suspected bowel perforation

PATIENT PREPARATION

- Usually none

SUPPLIES

- 1.0 mg glucagon
- 18 gauge needle (for drawing glucagon)
- 25 gauge needle (for injecting glucagon)
- 1 cc syringe (for glucagon)
- Tourniquet
- Alcohol swab
- Small bandage
- 500 cc barium (85% w/v) mixed into 1500 cc tepid water (to produce a 12–20% w/v solution)
- Barium enema bag
- Tubing-to-tubing adapter
- Single contrast enema tip with retention cuff (for Hartmann pouch exam)
- 10–18 Fr Foley catheter with 30 cc balloon, colostomy tip, or cone (for colostomy exam)
- 20 cc syringe (for inflating Foley balloon)
- Lubrication jelly
- ±Inflatable enema ring (if patient appears unable to retain contrast)
- Small towel

SCOUT FILM

- AP abdomen

SAMPLE DICTATION

A two-stage single contrast barium enema was performed for delineation of colonic anatomy prior to a colostomy takedown. This examination, performed on an unprepared bowel, is not sufficient for excluding small colonic lesions. The Hartmann pouch was filled to the stump located in the distal sigmoid colon. The second stage of the examination was performed through the colostomy site in the midleft abdomen. Barium filled the colon in a retrograde fashion from the descending colon to the cecum. The visualized colonic segments have a grossly unremarkable appearance. ■

RADIATION

- Fluoro: 750 mrad/min
- Spot films: 70 mrad per spot film

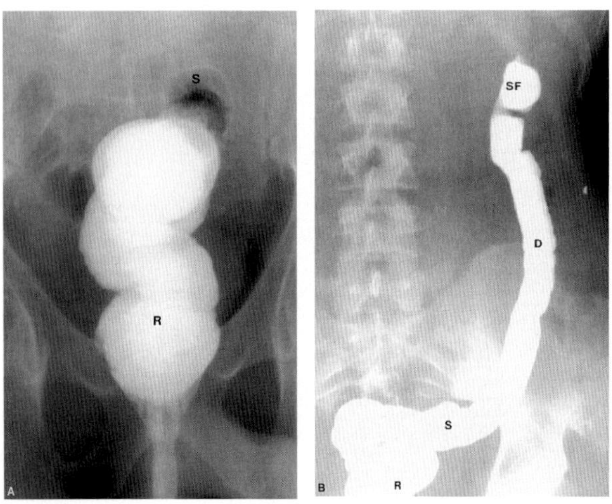

R—rectum
S—sigmoid
D—descending colon
SF—splenic flexure

FIGURE 1. *Various appearances of the Hartmann pouch, extending to the rectosigmoid junction (A) and the splenic flexure region (B).*

EXAM

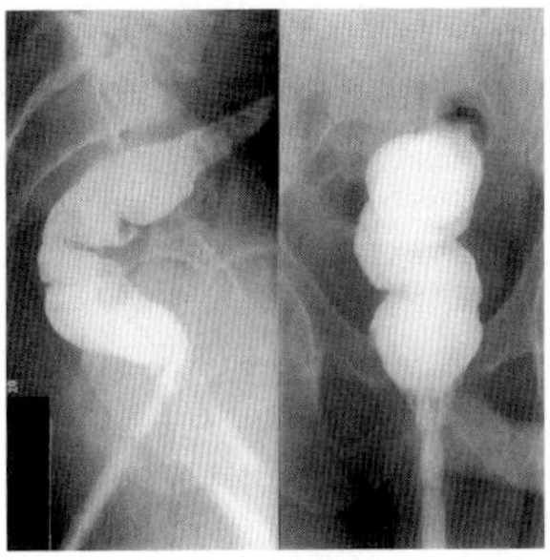

14 × 14
2 on 1
or
spot films

1 *Hartmann Pouch Exam*

In a multipart exam, the Hartmann pouch should be examined first. Contrast refluxed through the ileocecal valve during the colostomy exam can obscure the pouch.

With the patient in the Sims position, carefully place a lubricated single contrast enema tip in the rectum. Slowly distend the Hartmann pouch and image it in the following projections:

1. Lt Lat
2. AP
3. Oblique (if needed)

Continue filling until the end of the pouch is encountered, obtaining images as with a conventional single contrast barium enema. The Hartmann pouch may terminate in the rectosigmoid or may continue to the splenic flexure or beyond.

TABLETOP
Horizontal

110 kVp

PATIENT
Sims
Lt Lat
AP

℞

2 *Administer Glucagon*

If not contraindicated, administer 1.0 mg glucagon (intravenously if possible) prior to beginning the colostomy exam. Administer the glucagon slowly, as nausea and other side effects can result from rapid administration.

TABLETOP
Head Up
20–30°

PATIENT
AP

3a *Intubate Colostomy (Foley Catheter)*

The Foley catheter can be very effective if used properly. This method has been used thousands of times without incident and results in an easier, quicker, and cleaner exam. *The hazard of using a Foley catheter is that if it is not pushed far enough into the colon, inflation of the balloon can disrupt the site of attachment of the colon to the anterior abdominal wall. This could result in a colon perforation into the abdominal cavity, with serious results.*

Remove the colostomy bag and clean away any excess mucus and fecal material. Carefully examine the colostomy opening with a small finger to determine the direction of the colon. This will also indicate what size Foley catheter to use.

When inserting the catheter, make sure that it is several centimeters inside the colon before inflating the balloon. Gently inflate the balloon, then pull back gently to check for lodgement. If the balloon pulls out easily, try inflating with more air or use a larger catheter.

TABLETOP
Horizontal

PATIENT
AP

3b *Intubate Colostomy (Alternative)*

Alternatively, other devices, such as the suction cup, cone, or nipple, can be fitted over the colostomy site. A Foley catheter with a large balloon can also be externally pressed against the colostomy site.

TABLETOP
Horizontal

PATIENT
AP

4 *Fill Colostomy*

Connect the enema bag tubing to the Foley catheter with a large tubing connector and place a small towel over the colostomy site around the Foley catheter. Have the patient press on the towel to help prevent leakage of barium.

Do not hang the barium bag too high, as rapid filling of the colon can induce a vasovagal reaction.

TABLETOP
Horizontal

PATIENT
AP

5 *Image Entire Colon*

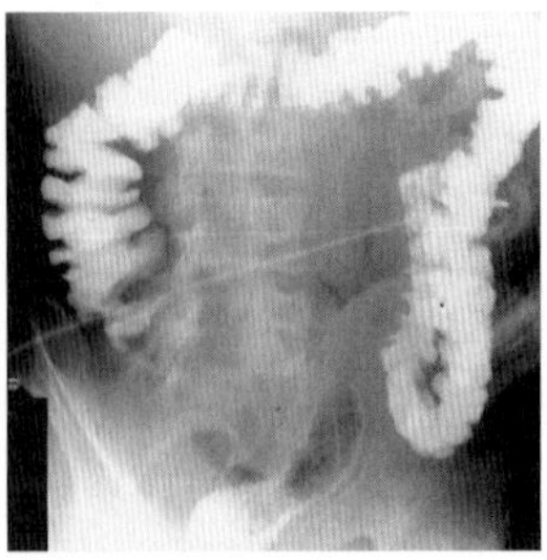

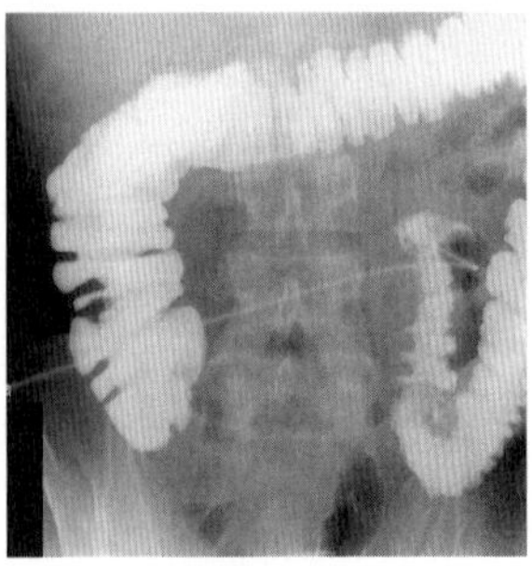

14 × 14
1 on 1

Use two or three 14 × 14 cassettes to image the entire colon.

Remember that the 14 × 14 cassettes will give a larger view than what appears on the monitor, so "cut off" some of the image on the monitor, as more will be seen on the film.

TABLETOP
Horizontal

PATIENT
AP
Various obliques

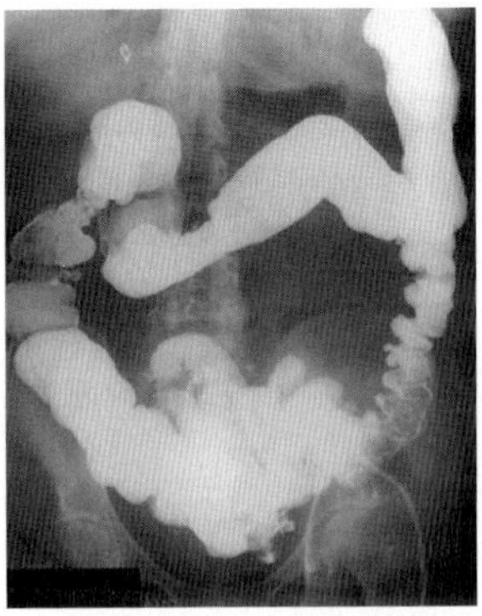

14 × 17

6 *Obtain Overhead Film*

Have the technologist obtain an overhead AP 14 × 17 film.

TABLETOP

Horizontal

90 kVp

PATIENT

AP

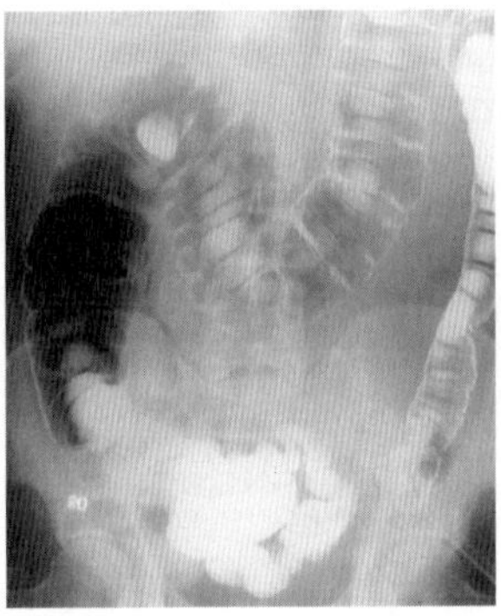

✪ *Double Contrast Colostomy Barium Enema*

Double contrast technique can also be used for evaluating the colon, particularly if the examination is being performed as a screening exam for colon cancer or for recurrence of tumor. This examination requires a prepared colon. Access the colostomy site as described above and complete the exam as for a routine double contrast barium enema. ■

Dynamic Proctography

INDICATIONS

- Difficulty with defecation
- Rectal prolapse

CONTRAINDICATIONS

- No common contraindications

PATIENT PREPARATION

- Some radiologists prefer to opacify the small bowel with 12–16 oz of 60% w/v barium 30 minutes prior to the exam, as well as to opacify the vagina in female patients with a tampon permeated with ~30% iodine water-soluble contrast.

SUPPLIES

- Cylinder of barium paste (100% w/v) (e.g., Evacu-Paste, Anatrast)
- Large-caliber flexible enema tip
- Lubrication jelly
- Caulking gun
- Brunswick chair (radiolucent commode)
- Plastic bag for the Brunswick chair basin (to collect evacuated barium paste)
- Gurney (for patient while instilling barium paste)

TABLE 1. *Dynamic Proctography Measurements*

MANEUVER	FEMALE	MALE
Neutral	70–134°	70–134°
Squeeze	64–108°	58–89°
Strain	75–108°	67–123°

SCOUT FILM

- Not obtained routinely

SAMPLE DICTATION

The rectum and distal sigmoid colon were filled with barium paste, and the patient was examined in the lateral sitting position. The anorectal angle measures 80° when squeezing, 105° when straining, and 95° in the neutral position. The measurements are all within normal limits. No anterior rectocele was identified. There was no significant residual after evacuation. ■

RADIATION

- Fluoro: 350 mrad/min
- Spot films: 25 mrad per spot film

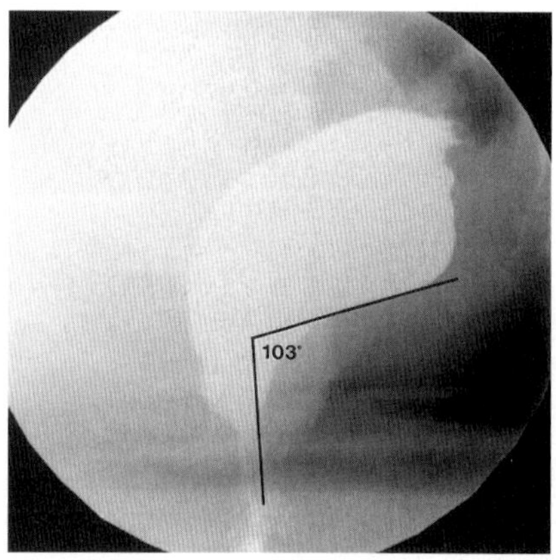

FIGURE 1. *Measurement of the anorectal angle.*

EXAM

1 *Explain Exam to Patient*

Obtain a short history from the patient regarding defecation problems. Explain the procedure with a description of the various maneuvers:

1. *Neutral* or relaxed
2. *Squeeze* or press-up
3. *Strain* without releasing
4. Strain with *evacuation*

Ascertain if the instructions are understood, and have the patient practice the maneuvers.

2 *Inject Contrast*

With a minimum number of staff present, place the patient in the Sims position on a gurney and carefully place the lubricated enema tip in the rectum. Inject barium paste, filling the rectum and sigmoid until the patient becomes slightly uncomfortable. This usually requires only about half of the tube.

TABLETOP
Vertical

PATIENT
Sims

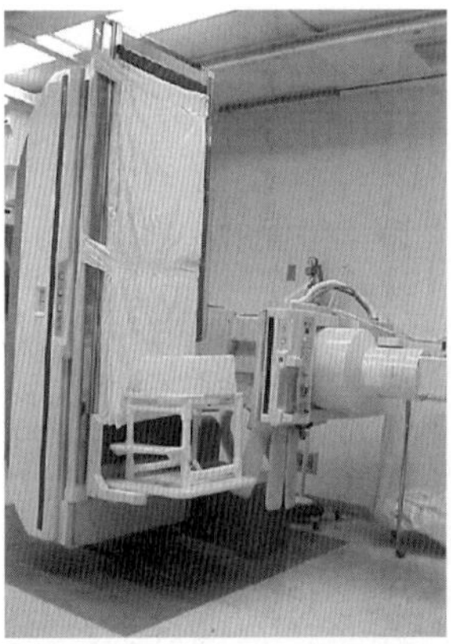

3 *Position Patient on Brunswick Chair*

Help the patient to the Brunswick chair, which is positioned between the fluoroscopy tabletop and the image intensifier. The Brunswick chair seat contains water, which eliminates the air gap that would degrade the image.

If the patient is unable to fit between the tabletop and the tower, a C-arm fluoroscope can be used.

TABLETOP
Vertical

PATIENT
Rt Lat

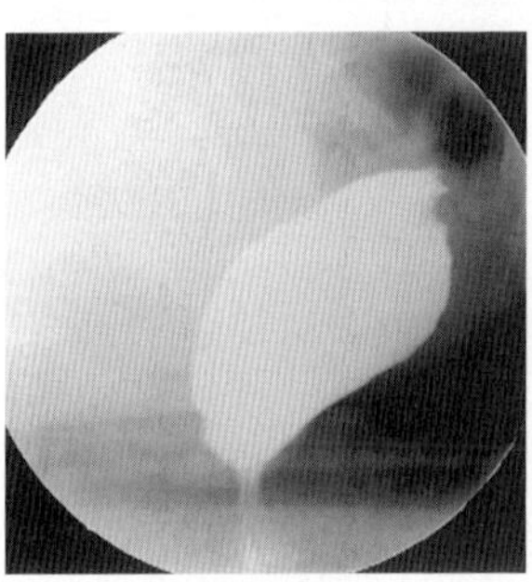

spot film

■▶

4 *Image "Neutral" Position*

Image the rectum in the "neutral" position, first with a spot film and then with the video recorder.

TABLETOP
Vertical

110 kVp

PATIENT
Rt Lat

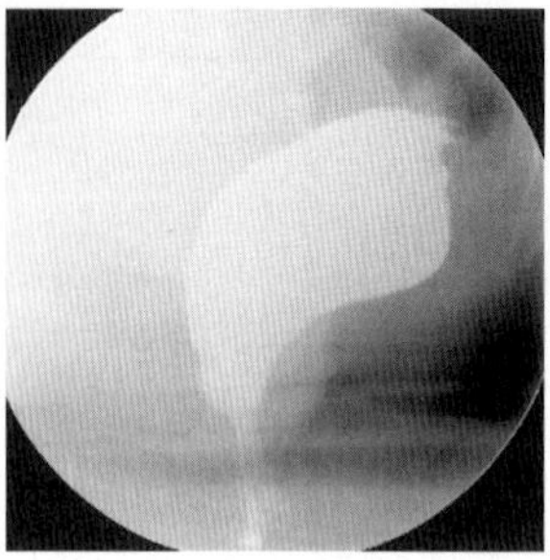

spot film

5 ***Image "Squeeze" Position***

Image the rectum in the "squeeze" position, first with a spot film and then with the video recorder.

TABLETOP

Vertical

PATIENT

Rt Lat

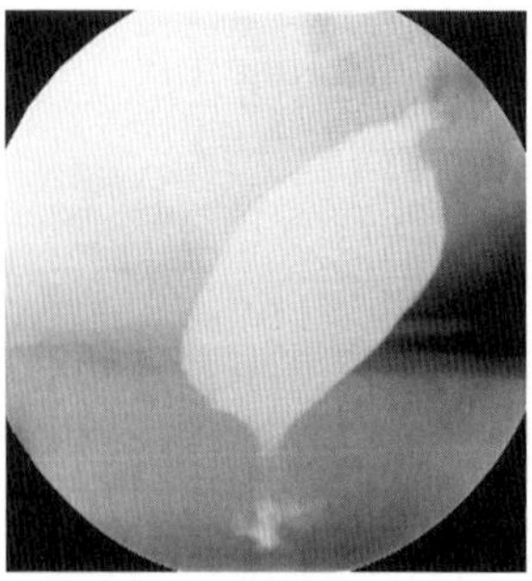

spot film

6 ***Image "Strain" Position***

Image the rectum in the "strain" position, first with a spot film and then with the video recorder.

TABLETOP

Vertical

PATIENT

Rt Lat

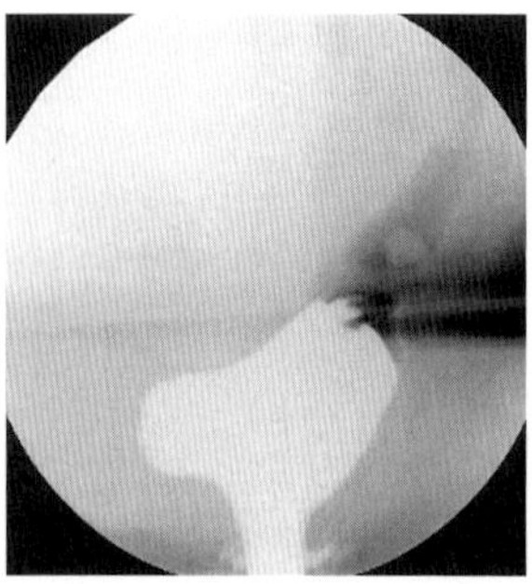

spot film

7 ***Image "Evacuation" Position***

Image the rectum in the "evacuation" position, first with a spot film and then with the video recorder.

TABLETOP

Vertical

PATIENT

Rt Lat

8 ***Measure Anorectal Angles***

After imaging, send the patient to the restroom to evacuate the remaining paste. Measure the anorectal angles on the spot films. ■

Colorectal Transit Exam

Although not a fluoroscopic procedure, the Colorectal Transit Exam is an occasionally encountered radiologic procedure that deserves inclusion.

INDICATIONS

- Chronic constipation

CONTRAINDICATIONS

- No common contraindications

PATIENT PREPARATION

- None

SUPPLIES

- 2 medicine cups (for capsule and water)
- One capsule containing 24 radiopaque polyvinyl chloride O-rings (e.g., Sitzmarks)
- 10 cc water

SAMPLE DICTATION

The patient ingested a single Sitzmarks capsule containing 24 radiopaque O-rings and returned for imaging after 5 days. The abdominal radiograph reveals that 21 (88%) of the markers have been eliminated. The 3 remaining markers project over the sigmoid colon. These findings are consistent with normal colonic transit. ■

RADIATION

- Spot films: 70 mrad per spot film

TABLE 1. *Number of Retained Markers (out of 24 total) Indicating the Percentage Expelled*

NORMAL	0 = 100%	1 = 96%	2 = 92%	3 = 88%	4 = 83%	5 = 79%
DELAYED	6 = 75%	7 = 71%	8 = 67%	9 = 63%	10 = 58%	11 = 54%
	12 = 50%	13 = 46%	14 = 43%	15 = 39%	16 = 33%	17 = 29%
TRANSIT	18 = 25%	19 = 21%	20 = 17%	21 = 13%	22 = 8%	23 = 4%

TABLE 2. *Interpretation of Abnormal Colonic Transit Exam*

FINDINGS	CONCLUSION
Markers scattered about colon	Likely colonic hypomotility or inertia
Markers accumulated in rectosigmoid	Likely functional outlet delay, such as internal rectal prolapse or anismus

EXAM

1 Have Patient Swallow Capsule

On day 0, the patient swallows a single capsule with water under medical observation. The patient is instructed not to use enemas, laxatives, or suppositories for 5 days.

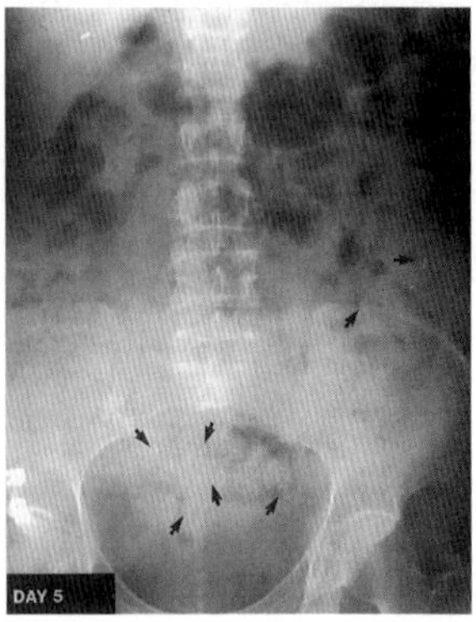

14 × 17

2 Count Retained Markers

On day 5, the patient returns for an AP abdominal radiograph. The markers are counted, and the percentage of expelled markers is calculated:

$$\% \text{ expelled markers} = \frac{24 - (\text{visualized markers})}{24}$$

Normal colonic transit is indicated if the patient has expelled ~80% of the markers.

TABLETOP

Horizontal

75 kVp

PATIENT

AP

3 Follow-Up Exam (If Required)

If less than 20% of the markers were expelled, the patient is instructed to take a stool bulking agent daily for 1–2 weeks, after which the exam is repeated. ■

PART IV
Biliary Examinations

Jeffrey D. Houston, M.D.
Michael Davis, M.D.

T-Tube Cholangiogram

Oral Cholecystogram

Endoscopic Retrograde Cholangiopancreatogram

T-Tube Cholangiogram

INDICATIONS

- Evaluation for retained biliary calculi
- Assessment for postoperative bile leak
- Delineation of bilary ductal anatomy

CONTRAINDICATIONS

- No common contraindications

PATIENT PREPARATION

- None

SUPPLIES

- 20 cc 30–40% iodine water-soluble intravascular contrast (e.g., Hypaque-76, MD-76, RenoCal-76)
- 20 cc syringe (for contrast)
- 18 gauge needle (for drawing contrast)
- 2 povidone-iodine swabs
- 21 gauge butterfly needle and tubing
- Sterile 4 × 4 gauze
- Hemostat

SCOUT FILM

- AP abdomen

SAMPLE DICTATION

Under fluoroscopic guidance, 14 cc RenoCal-76 was injected through the patient's existing T-tube, with resulting opacification of the entire biliary system. Both the extrahepatic and intrahepatic biliary systems are normal in caliber, without evidence of strictures, filling defects, or extrinsic masses. Free spillage of contrast into the duodenum was observed. ■

RADIATION

- Fluoro: 650 mrad/min
- Spot films: 50 mrad per spot film

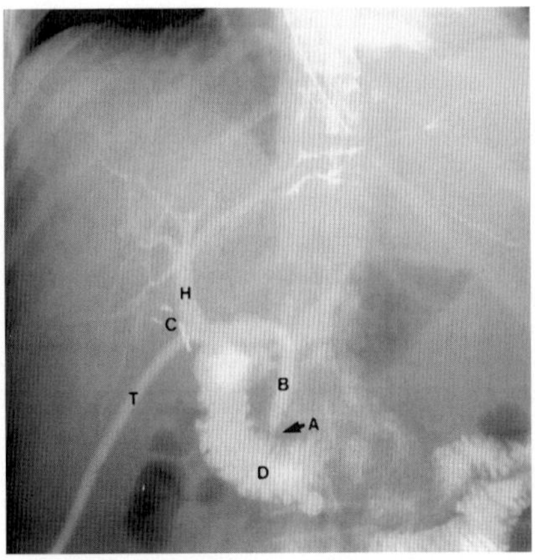

H—**common hepatic duct**
T—**T-tube (extending through cystic duct remnant)**
C—**cholecystectomy clips**
B—**common bile duct**
A—**ampulla of Vater**
D—**duodenum**

FIGURE 1. *Postcholecystectomy anatomy of the biliary system.*

EXAM

1 Prepare Tubing

Attach the 21 gauge butterfly needle to the 20 cc syringe and flush the tubing with contrast to expel all of the air.

2 Cleanse T-Tube Injection Site

Clamp the T-tube a few centimeters from the abdominal wall with the hemostat. Cleanse a selected site on the T-tube proximal to the hemostat twice with povidone-iodine swabs. Then wipe off the excess povidone-iodine with sterile 4 × 4 gauze.

TABLETOP
Horizontal

PATIENT
AP

3 Eliminate Air Bubbles in Contrast

With the butterfly needle in hand, have the technologist push a small amount of contrast out of the tip of the needle and then insert it into the T-tube. Once the lumen is reached, advance the needle parallel to the lumen until it is secured. Withdraw the plunger and observe the fluid in the butterfly tubing. If bile is present without air bubbles, proceed with the procedure, ensuring that any filling defects seen in the biliary system are not introduced bubbles.

TABLETOP
Horizontal

PATIENT
AP

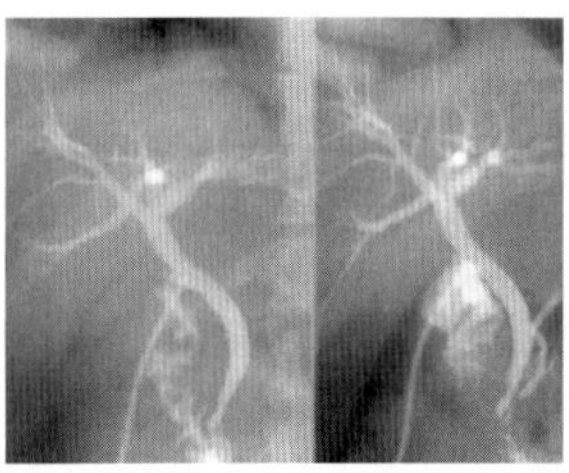

10 × 12
2 on 1
or
spot film
mag

4 Image Biliary Ductal Segments

Bring the fluoroscope into place, being careful not to dislodge the needle. Under fluoroscopic guidance, inject contrast with gentle pressure until the bile ducts begin to opacify. When the biliary system is adequately distended, obtain the following images:

1. Common hepatic duct
2. Common bile duct
3. Intrahepatic ducts
4. Spillage of contrast into the duodenum

TABLETOP
Horizontal

75 kVp

PATIENT
AP
±RPO

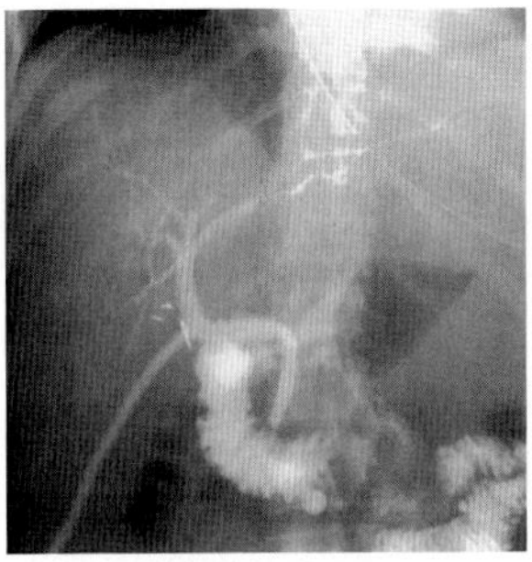

14 × 14
1 on 1

5 *Film Entire Biliary System*

Lastly, use a 14 × 14 cassette to film the entire biliary system. View the developed films *before* disconnecting the needle and unclamping the tube. ■

TABLETOP
Horizontal

PATIENT
AP
±RPO

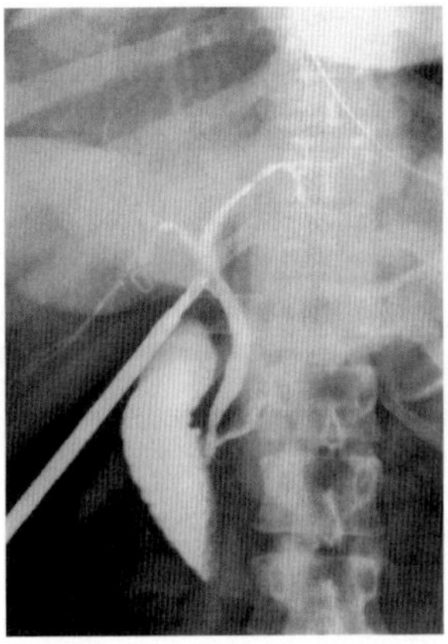

✪ *Intraoperative Cholangiogram*

Intraoperative cholangiograms can be imaged in the same fashion as T-tube cholangiograms, except that the surgeon directly injects the contrast through the cystic duct remnant. ■

TABLETOP
Horizontal

75 kVp

PATIENT
AP
±RPO

Oral Cholecystogram

INDICATIONS

- Inadequate sonographic evaluation of gallbladder for cholelithiasis
- Persistent unexplained right upper quadrant pain

CONTRAINDICATIONS

- Renal insufficiency (BUN >30, Cr >1.5)
- Liver insufficiency
- Prior allergic reaction to contrast agent

PATIENT PREPARATION

- AP abdominal film prior to administering contrast agent
- NPO after midnight or 6 hours prior to exam
- Six 0.5 g tablets iopanoic acid (Telepaque) or tyropanoate sodium (Bilopaque) at 6:00 P.M. with a meal on 2 consecutive days before the exam, to prevent the patient from having to return the following day after repeating the dose if the gallbladder was poorly visualized after one dose. Inpatients may receive a single 3 g dose the night before the exam.

SUPPLIES

- ± 0.02 to 0.04 μg/kg sincalide (Kinevac)
- $\pm$3 cc syringe (for sincalide)
- $\pm$25 gauge needle (for sincalide)
- $\pm$Tourniquet
- $\pm$Alcohol swab

SCOUT FILM

- Not obtained routinely

SAMPLE DICTATION

Oral cholecystography was performed utilizing two 3 g doses of Telepaque. There is complete opacification of the gallbladder, which has a normal appearance. There is no evidence of cholelithiasis or any other significant abnormality. ■

RADIATION

- Fluoro: 650 mrad/min
- Spot films: 50 mrad per spot film

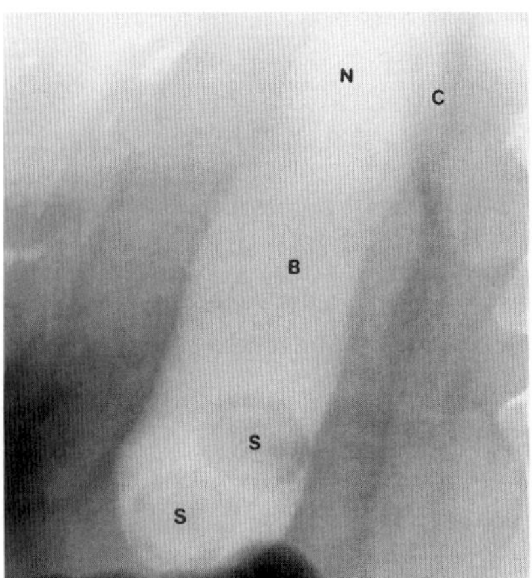

C—cystic duct
N—neck
B—body (corpus)
F—fundus
S—stone

FIGURE 1. *Anatomy of the gallbladder.*

EXAM

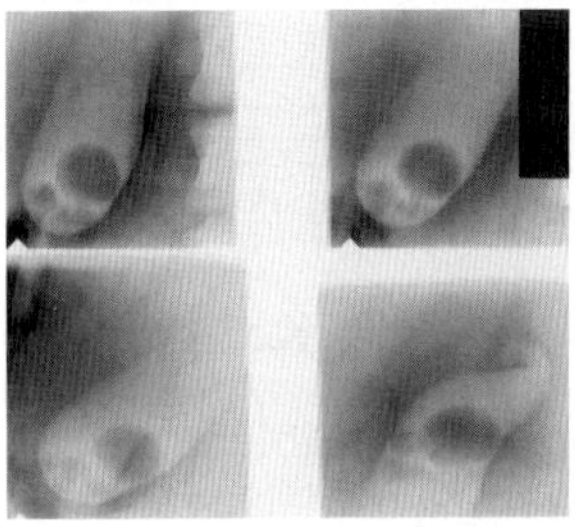

10 × 12
4 on 1
or
spot film

1 *Image Gallbladder in Erect and Head-Down Positions*

With the patient standing on the footboard, locate the gallbladder fluoroscopically. Obtain AP and RPO views of the gallbladder in the upright position, then obtain the same images after declining the tabletop to −30°. These views of the gallbladder are obtained to ensure filling of the gallbladder neck. The compression cone may be used to displace overlying bowel.

If the gallbladder is insufficiently visualized, the exam can be repeated the following day after administration of a second dose of contrast. If an outpatient has received two consecutive doses, the exam is considered complete.

TABLETOP
Vertical →
Head Down
−30°

75 kVp

PATIENT
AP
RPO

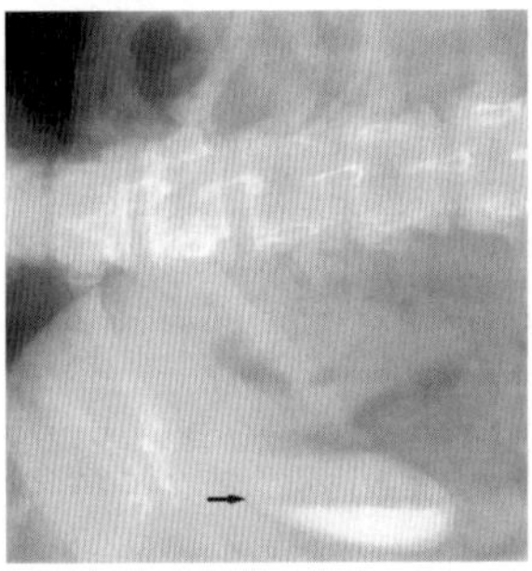

10 × 12

2 *Film Right Lateral Decubitus Gallbladder*

Have the technologist obtain a right lateral decubitus film centered over the lateral border of the gallbladder.

Bile, calculi, and contrast will layer based on their respective densities.

TABLETOP
Horizontal

75 kVp

PATIENT
Rt Lat

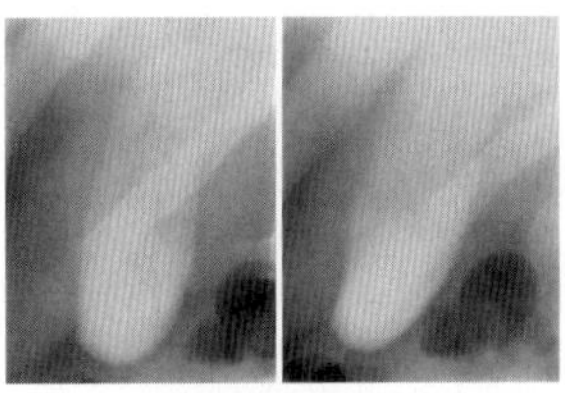

10 × 12
2 on 1
or
spot film

3 *Obtain Postprandial Film (if Requested)*

An assessment of gallbladder emptying is rarely requested, but can be performed by obtaining additional erect AP and RPO films 20–40 minutes after stimulation of the gallbladder with a fatty meal or 5–15 minutes after sincalide administration (0.02 μg /kg). If not contraindicated, sincalide should be intravenously administered over 30–60 seconds, as a rapid bolus can produce abdominal pain, nausea, and spasm of the gallbladder neck. A second dose of sincalide (0.04 μg/kg) can be administered at 15 minutes if the initial response was unsatisfactory. ■

TABLETOP
Vertical

PATIENT
AP
RPO

Endoscopic Retrograde Cholangiopancreatogram

INDICATIONS

- Choledocholithiasis
- Biliary obstruction
- Suspicion of variant biliary ductal anatomy
- Recurrent pancreatitis
- Pancreatic malignancy

CONTRAINDICATIONS

- Contraindications to upper gastrointestinal endoscopy
- Suppurative cholangitis
- Acute pancreatitis (relative contraindication)
- Pancreatic pseudocysts (relative contraindication)

PATIENT PREPARATION

- NPO after midnight
- Premedication if there is a history of prior reactions to contrast

SUPPLIES

- 20+ cc ~30% iodine water-soluble intravascular contrast (e.g., Hypaque Meglumine 60%, Reno-60, Conray)
- Supplies for endoscopic procedure per endoscopist

SCOUT FILM

- Not obtained routinely

SAMPLE DICTATION

After endoscopic cannulation, sequential imaging of the biliary and pancreatic ductal systems was performed, using 17 cc Reno-60. The bile and pancreatic ducts are all normal in caliber, without evidence of strictures, external mass effect, filling defects, or extravasation. ■

Radiation

- Fluoro: 650 mrad/min
- Spot films: 50 mrad per spot film

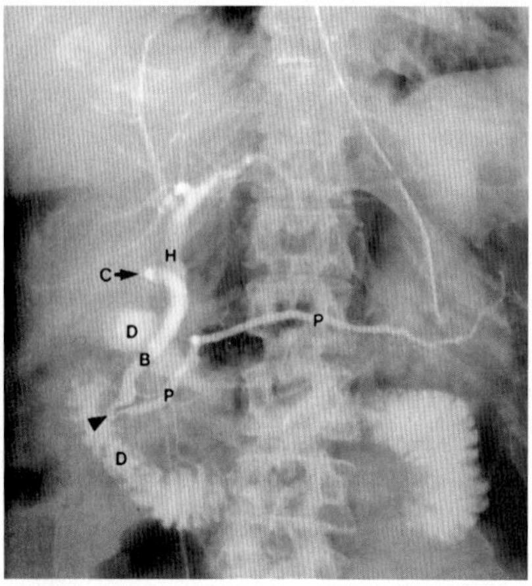

H—common hepatic duct
C—cystic duct (remnant)
B—common bile duct
arrowhead—major papilla and ampulla of Vater
P—main pancreatic duct
D—duodenum

FIGURE 1. *Normal biliary and pancreatic ductal anatomy, as delineated by an intraoperative cholangiogram (from Mettler FA:* Essentials of Radiology. *Philadelphia, W.B. Saunders, 1996, p. 200).*

EXAM

1 *Cannulation of Major Papilla by Endoscopist*

Endoscopic retrograde cholangiopancreatography (ERCP) is now performed primarily by gastroenterologists, with the images subsequently provided for radiologic interpretation. At some institutions, radiologists actively participate in the image acquisition process. Using conscious patient sedation, the endoscopist will cannulate the major papilla, which can be relaxed with 0.5 mg intravenous glucagon.

TABLETOP
Horizontal

PATIENT
Various

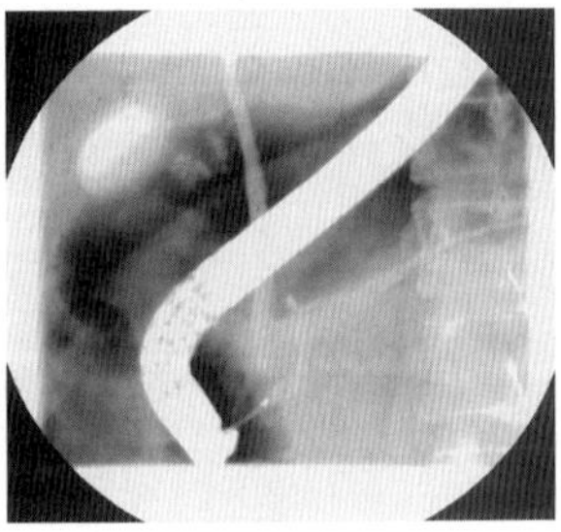

spot film
or
10 × 12
1 on 1

2 *Inject Contrast*

Under fluoroscopic visualization, the endoscopist slowly injects contrast to gradually opacify the ductal system. Early sequential imaging and close observation for air bubbles (which can mimic calculi) are essential.

Full-strength contrast is generally used for the pancreatic duct, whereas diluted contrast is commonly employed to opacify the larger bile ducts, especially in a patulous system. Filling with overly dense contrast creates the risk of missing small filling defects.

Occasionally, it is possible to fill both the pancreatic duct and the bile ducts with a single injection, but it is often necessary to cannulate each ductal system selectively. As the common bile duct is difficult to cannulate once the pancreatic duct is filled, the pancreatic duct is commonly imaged first.

TABLETOP
Horizontal

75 kVp

PATIENT
Various

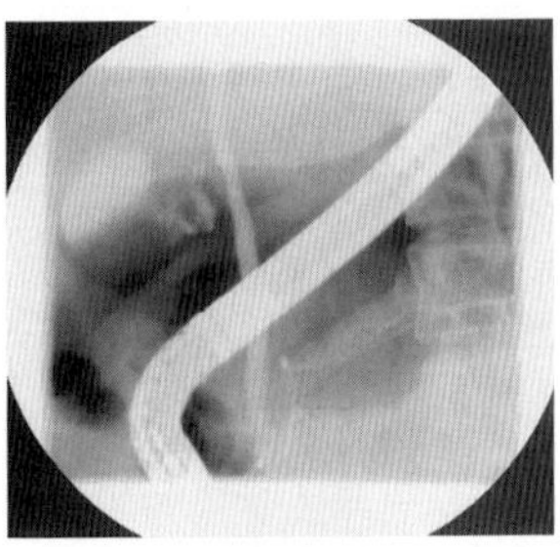

spot film
or
10 × 12
1 on 1

3 *Image Pancreatogram*

Obtain spot films as the pancreatic duct is filled with contrast (2–4 cc is suitable for most cases). It is optimal to fill the small side branches, but acinarization should be avoided, as overfilling is associated with an increased risk of post-ERCP pancreatitis.

As the distal pancreatic duct is directed posteriorly, it can be difficult to fill the tail segment. To facilitate filling of the entire pancreatic duct, the patient can be turned to the LAO position.

TABLETOP
Horizontal

PATIENT
Various

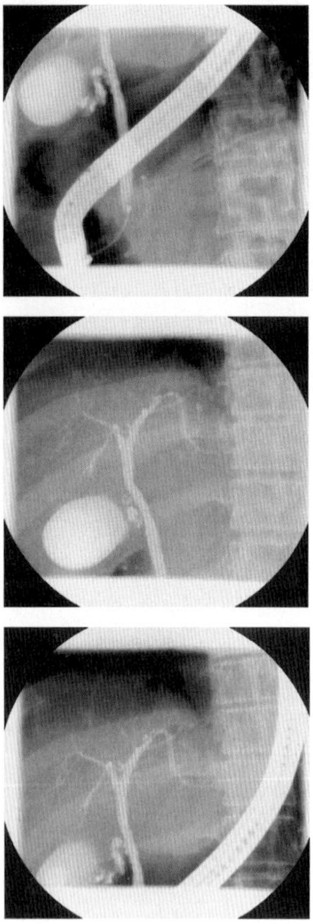

spot film
or
10 × 12
1 on 1

4 *Image Cholangiogram*

Obtain spot films to document complete filling of the biliary tree, including:

1. Common bile duct
2. Cystic duct and gallbladder (if present)
3. Common hepatic duct
4. Intrahepatic ducts

In the prone position, the more anterior left intrahepatic ductal system will fill preferentially. Filling of the right intrahepatic ductal system can be facilitated by supine positioning.

Proximal intrahepatic ducts are preferentially filled by elevating the tabletop, whereas distal common bile duct visualization can be improved by declining the head of the tabletop. ■

TABLETOP
Horizontal

PATIENT
Various

PART V

Genitourinary Examinations

Jeffrey D. Houston, M.D.
Michael Davis, M.D.

Cystogram

Voiding Cystourethrogram

Retrograde Urethrogram

Loop-o-Gram/Pouch-o-Gram

Fluoroscopic Intravenous Urogram

Nephrostogram

Hysterosalpingogram

Cystogram

INDICATIONS

- Assessment of vesicoureteral reflux
- Suspected bladder rupture
- Definition of bladder anatomy
- Determination of postvoid residual

CONTRAINDICATIONS

- Possible urethral injury (exam should be preceded by a retrograde urethrogram)

PATIENT PREPARATION

- None

SUPPLIES

- 500+ cc 8% iodine water-soluble uroradiologic contrast (e.g., Cysto-Conray II, Cystografin Dilute)
- Plastic tubing with flow control device
- Luer to catheter tubing adapter
- 18 gauge needle (to vent contrast bottle)
- 8–10 Fr Foley catheter
- 2% viscous lidocaine gel
- Sterile gloves (latex-free if latex allergy/precautions)
- Sterile drape (± fenestration, depending on gender of patient)
- Povidone-iodine solution (e.g., Betadine)
- Sterile cotton balls
- Basin (to collect residual urine)
- Cloth tape
- Disposable urinal

SCOUT FILM

- AP pelvis

SAMPLE DICTATION

An 8 Fr Foley catheter was placed through the urethra, and the urinary bladder was filled with 350 cc Cystografin Dilute by gravity. The bladder is normal in size and has normal contours. No filling defects are identified. There was no vesicoureteral reflux or significant postvoid residual. ■

RADIATION

- Fluoro: 400 mrad/min
- Spot films: 40 mrad per spot film

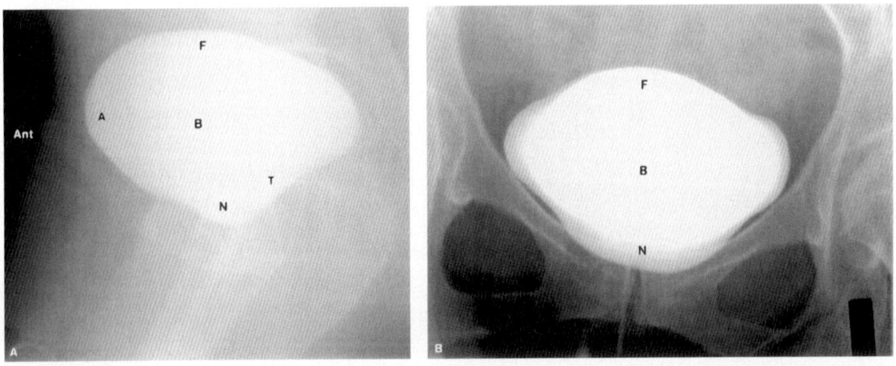

F—fundus
A—apex
B—body (corpus)
T—trigone
N—neck

FIGURE 1. Normal bladder anatomy in lateral (A) and AP (B) projections.

EXAM

℞

1 Catheterize Urinary Bladder

Using sterile technique, catheterize the urinary bladder with a Foley catheter that is lubricated with lidocaine gel. Drain any residual urine from the bladder so that it does not dilute the contrast. It is usually not necessary to inflate the catheter balloon. Secure the catheter to the patient's skin using a small amount of tape.

TABLETOP
Horizontal

PATIENT
AP

2 Instill Contrast

Connect the contrast-primed tubing to the catheter and begin filling by gravity. Ask the patient to inform you when there is a significant need to void. Record the amount of contrast administered.

If contrast begins to leak around the catheter, the balloon can be inflated and light traction applied to the catheter to mechanically obstruct the bladder neck.

If orthopedic hardware (such as a pelvic fixator) prohibits movement of the image intensifier over the patient, instill 100 cc contrast by gravity and obtain an overhead AP film. If there is no evidence of extravasation, fill with another 150 cc contrast by gravity and obtain overhead films.

TABLETOP
Horizontal

75 kVp

PATIENT
AP

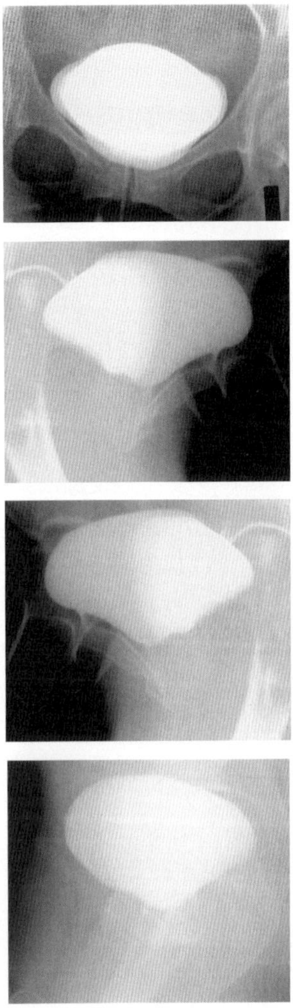

10 × 12
1 on 1
or
spot film

3 Film Bladder

Film the urinary bladder in the following positions:

1. AP
2. RPO
3. LPO
4. Rt Lat

TABLETOP
Horizontal

PATIENT
AP
RPO
LPO
Rt Lat

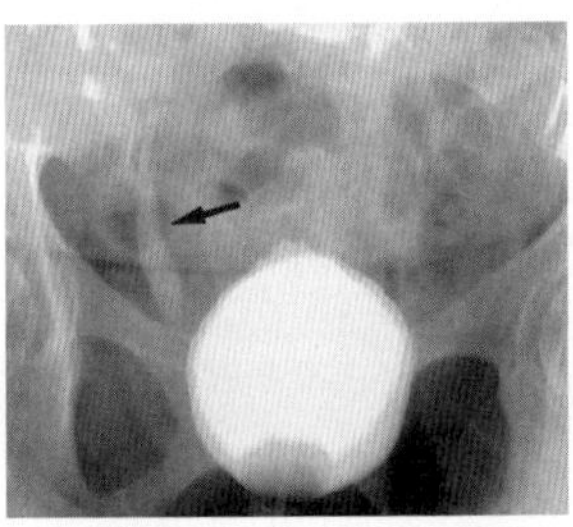

10 × 12
1 on 1
or
spot film

4 Assess for Vesicoureteral Reflux

Visualize the bladder and observe for vesicoureteral reflux. Obtain films if reflux is seen, documenting the most superior extent of the reflux.

TABLETOP
Horizontal

PATIENT
AP

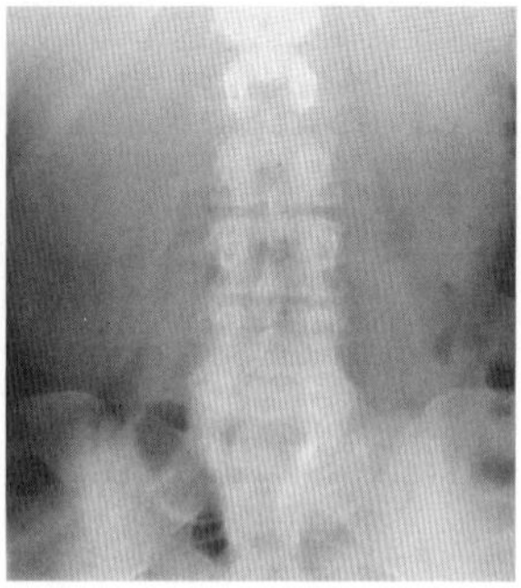

14 × 14
1 on 1
or
spot film

5 *Film Kidneys*

Image each kidney, looking for the presence of contrast from vesicoureteral reflux.

TABLETOP
Horizontal

PATIENT
AP

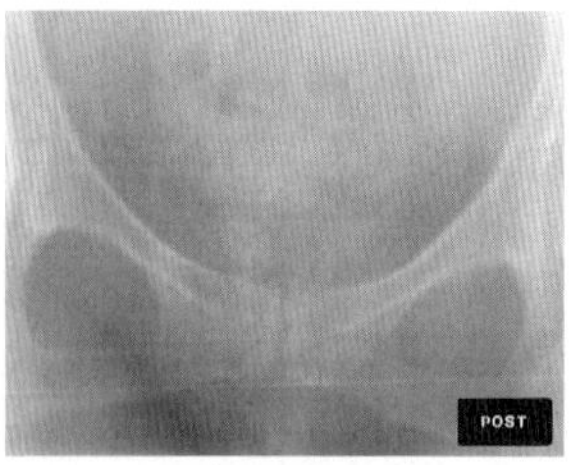

10 × 12
1 on 1
or
spot film

6 *Film Postvoid Bladder*

Send the patient to the restroom with a disposable urinal to void to completion. Obtain one image of the postvoid bladder. Calculate the postvoid residual (PVR):

PVR = (contrast instilled) − (contrast voided) ■

TABLETOP
Horizontal

PATIENT
AP

Voiding Cystourethrogram

INDICATIONS

- Assessment for vesicoureteral reflux
- Definition of urethral anatomy

CONTRAINDICATIONS

- Possible urethral injury (exam should be preceded by a retrograde urethrogram)

PATIENT PREPARATION

- None

SUPPLIES

- 500+ cc 8% iodine water-soluble uroradiologic contrast (e.g., Cysto-Conray II, Cystografin Dilute)
- Plastic tubing with flow control device
- Luer to catheter tubing adapter
- 18 gauge needle (to vent contrast bottle)
- 8–10 Fr Foley catheter
- 2% viscous lidocaine gel
- Sterile gloves (latex-free if latex allergy/precautions)
- Sterile drape (± fenestration, depending on gender of patient)
- Povidone-iodine solution (e.g., Betadine)
- Sterile cotton balls
- Basin (to collect residual urine)
- Cloth tape
- Disposable urinal

SCOUT FILM

- AP pelvis

SAMPLE DICTATION

An 8 Fr Foley catheter was placed through the urethra, and the urinary bladder was filled with 350 cc Cystografin Dilute by gravity. The bladder is normal in size and has normal contours. No filling defects are identified. Voiding images reveal a normal-appearing urethra. There was no vesicoureteral reflux or significant postvoid residual. ■

RADIATION

- Fluoro: 400 mrad/min
- Spot films: 40 mrad per spot film

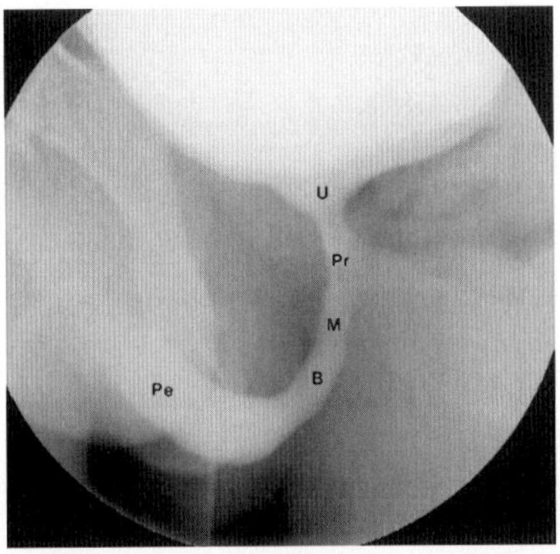

U—uvula of bladder
Pr—prostatic urethra
M—membranous urethra
B—bulbous urethra
Pe—pendulous urethra

FIGURE 1. *Normal urethral anatomy.*

EXAM

1–5 *Obtain Cystogram* *(see p. 105)*

Perform steps 1 through 5 of a routine cystogram, obtaining AP, LPO, RPO, and lateral views of the distended bladder, as well as assessing for vesicoureteral reflux.

TABLETOP
Horizontal

75 kVp

6 *Position Patient for Urethrogram*

Remove the catheter and bring the tabletop to the vertical position. If the patient is male, have him turn RPO, with the right thigh forward and the left thigh extended backward (to decrease the mass effect of the thighs and improve visualization of the urethra). Give a disposable urinal to the patient. Female patients should be directed to hold the urinal between their thighs, thus keeping their hands out of the field of view.

PATIENT
AP

TABLETOP
Vertical

PATIENT
♂RPO
♀AP

7 *Image Urethra*

Position the fluoroscope so that the base of the bladder can be seen; then ask the patient to void. As the urethra fills with contrast, begin imaging. Image the entire urethra.

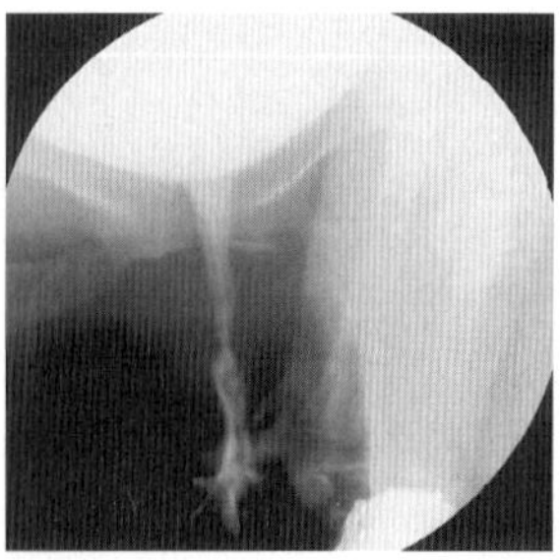

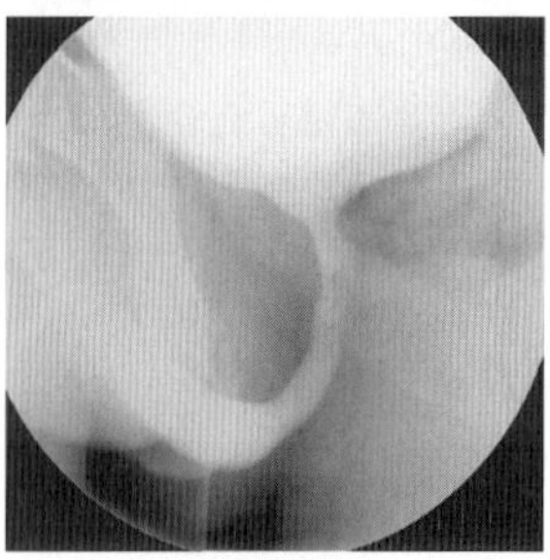

spot film
mag
or
10 × 12
1–2 on 1

TABLETOP
Vertical

rapid seq
2 fr/sec

PATIENT
♂RPO
♀AP

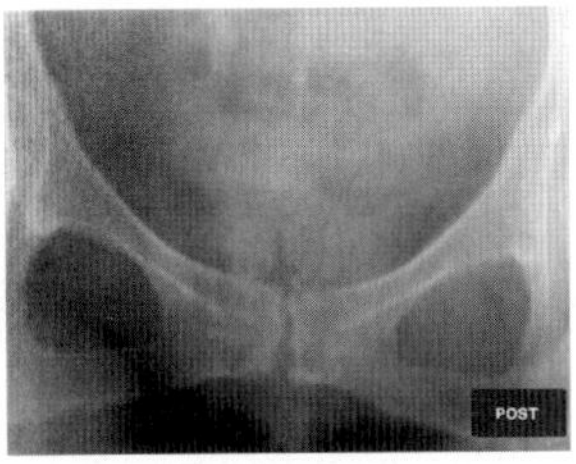

10 × 12
1 on 1
or
spot film

8 *Film Postvoid Bladder*

Obtain one image of the postvoid bladder. Calculate the postvoid residual (PVR):

PVR = (contrast instilled) − (contrast voided) ■

TABLETOP
Vertical

PATIENT
AP

Retrograde Urethrogram

INDICATIONS

- Definition of urethral anatomy
- Evaluation of urethral strictures and fistulas
- Urethral trauma

CONTRAINDICATIONS

- No common contraindications

PATIENT PREPARATION

- None

SUPPLIES

- 8–10 Fr Foley catheter with 3 cc balloon
- 20 cc 30–40% iodine water-soluble intravascular contrast (e.g., Hypaque-76, MD-76, RenoCal-76)
- 20 cc syringe (for contrast)
- Luer to catheter tubing adapter
- 18 gauge needle (for drawing contrast)
- 3 cc syringe (for inflating balloon)
- 2 povidone-iodine swabs
- 2% viscous lidocaine gel
- Sterile fenestrated drape
- Sterile 4 × 4 gauze
- Sterile gloves (latex-free if latex allergy/precautions)

SCOUT FILM

- Not obtained routinely

SAMPLE DICTATION

The urethra was filled with RenoCal-76 in a retrograde fashion through an 8 Fr Foley catheter placed in the navicular fossa. The urethral lumen is normal in size. No strictures or filling defects are identified. ■

RADIATION

- Fluoro: 400 mrad/min
- Spot films: 40 mrad per spot film

TABLE 1. *Types of Urethral Injuries*

TYPE	DESCRIPTION
1	Urethra is intact but elongated and narrowed by a periurethral hematoma
2	Partial or complete urethral disruption above the urogenital diaphragm with extraperitoneal contrast extravasation
3	Complete urethral disruption at the urogenital diaphragm with extraperitoneal and perineal contrast extravasation

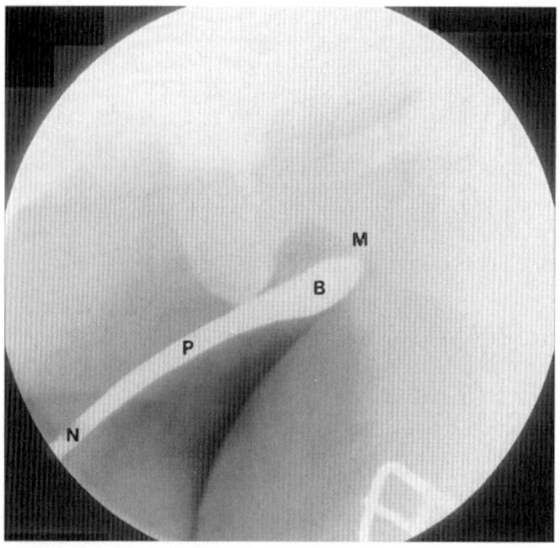

N—navicular fossa containing balloon
P—pendulous urethra
B—bulbous urethra
M—membranous urethra

FIGURE 1. *Urethral anatomy. Occasionally, the prostatic urethra and bladder cannot be opacified.*

EXAM

1 *Prepare Catheter* Using sterile technique, connect the syringe filled with contrast to the Foley catheter and fill the lumen to express the air from the catheter. Connect an inflated 3 cc syringe to the air inlet of the Foley catheter and inject 2.5 cc air to verify that the balloon inflates properly; then deflate the balloon.	
2 *Apply Sterile Drape* Cover the genital area with a sterile drape, with the penis extending through the fenestration.	***TABLETOP*** Horizontal ***PATIENT*** RPO
3 *Cleanse Meatus* Cleanse the perimeatal region with each of two povidone-iodine swabs; then wipe with sterile 4 × 4 gauze.	***TABLETOP*** Horizontal ***PATIENT*** RPO
4 *Catheterize Navicular Fossa* Put a small amount of lidocaine gel on the tip of the catheter and insert it about 2 cm into the urethra so that the balloon is in the navicular fossa. Then cautiously inflate the balloon with 2–3 cc air while rotating the catheter. After the balloon becomes lodged, disconnect the syringe. *Avoid overinflating the balloon, which could rupture the urethra.*	***TABLETOP*** Horizontal ***PATIENT*** RPO
5 *Apply Tourniquet* Unfold a dampened 4 × 4 gauze and then refold it in half longitudinally to use as a tourniquet. Place the tourniquet around the glans penis to encompass the balloon and twist until it is moderately tight. This will keep the balloon in place and will allow for traction to elongate the urethra for better visualization.	***TABLETOP*** Horizontal ***PATIENT*** RPO

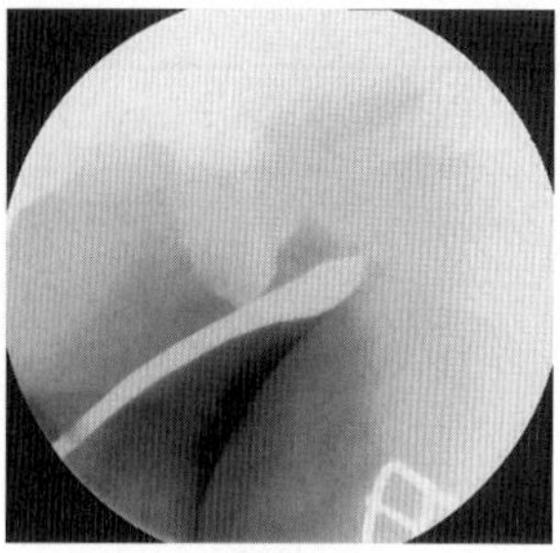

spot film
mag
or
10 × 12
2 on 1

6 *Film Urethra*

With the patient in the RPO position and while observing under fluoroscopy, slowly fill the urethra with contrast. Obtain images of the entire urethra. Avoid overdistending the urethra, which could result in rupture.

It is common for contrast not to flow beyond the membranous urethra. Sometimes contrast can be passed into the bladder by having the patient consciously try to relax the pelvic muscles.

If there is suspicion of a distal urethral stricture, have the technologist deflate the balloon so the radiologist can simultaneously image the distal urethra as the balloon is expelled.

TABLETOP
Horizontal

75 kVp

PATIENT
RPO

7 *Withdraw Contrast and Remove Catheter*

When imaging is complete, withdraw the contrast into the syringe. Do not remove the catheter until the images are deemed satisfactory; then deflate the balloon and remove the catheter. ■

TABLETOP
Horizontal

PATIENT
RPO

Loop-o-Gram/Pouch-o-Gram

INDICATIONS

- Evaluation of urinary diversion procedure

CONTRAINDICATIONS

- No common contraindications

PATIENT PREPARATION

- None

SUPPLIES

- 500+ cc 8% iodine uroradiologic contrast (e.g., Cysto-Conray II, Cystografin Dilute)
- Plastic tubing with flow control device
- 18 gauge needle (to vent contrast bottle)
- Luer to catheter tubing adapter
- Assortment of Foley catheters with 3 cc balloons
- 3 cc syringe (for inflating balloon)

SCOUT FILM

- AP abdomen

SAMPLE DICTATION

After placement of a 10 Fr Foley catheter through the ileostomy site into the neobladder, the system was filled with Cystografin Dilute by gravity. Normal reflux into both ureters and the renal collecting systems was seen. The collecting systems of both kidneys are dilated, but there is no evidence of obstruction. ■

RADIATION

- Fluoro: 600 mrad/min
- Spot films: 40 mrad per spot film

EXAM

1 *Catheterize Ileostomy*

Identify the ileostomy site and determine the Foley catheter size needed. Place the catheter well into the site and inflate the balloon cautiously then gently retract the catheter to test for secure placement. Connect the catheter to the plastic tubing and begin filling with contrast by gravity.

TABLETOP
Horizontal

PATIENT
AP

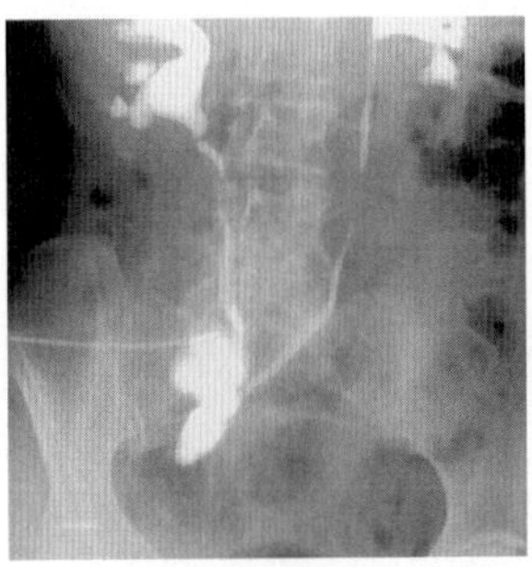

14 × 14
1 on 1
or
spot film

2 *Image Entire System*

Obtain images as the system fills, stopping after images of the filled collecting systems become completely opacified.

TABLETOP
Horizontal

75 kVp

PATIENT
AP

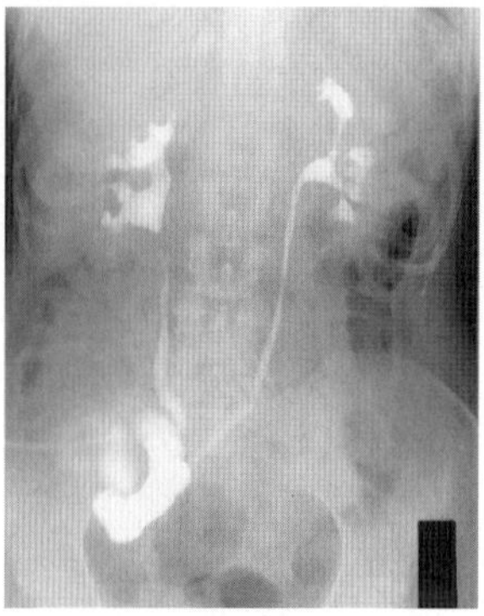

14 × 17

3 *Obtain Overhead Film*

Have the technologist obtain an overhead AP 14 × 17 film.

TABLETOP
Horizontal

75 kVp

PATIENT
AP

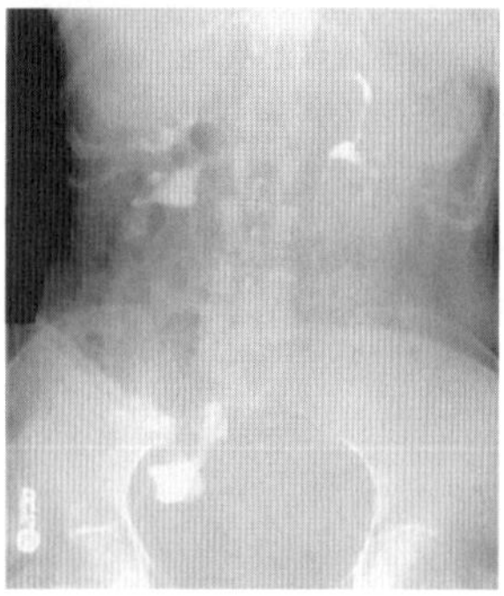

14 × 17

4 *Obtain Postdrainage Film*

After the images have been viewed and are deemed satisfactory, place the bottle of contrast on the floor and drain the system. Have the technologist obtain an overhead AP 14 × 17 postdrainage film. ■

TABLETOP
Horizontal

75 kVp

PATIENT
AP

Fluoroscopic Intravenous Urogram

INDICATIONS

- Evaluation of urolithiasis
- Visualization of ureteral or collecting system abnormalities

CONTRAINDICATIONS

- Renal insufficiency (BUN > 30, Cr > 1.5)
- Metformin (Glucophage) should be temporarily discontinued for 48 hours following the exam because of the risk of lactic acidosis and reinstated only after reassessment of renal function
- Severe prior contrast reaction

PATIENT PREPARATION

- Premedication if there is a history of prior contrast reactions
- 12 oz magnesium citrate at 6:00 P.M. on the day prior to the exam
- NPO after midnight

SUPPLIES

- ±Written consent form
- 100 cc 30% iodine nonionic intravascular contrast (e.g., Isovue-300, Omnipaque-300, Optiray 300, Oxilan 300, Ultravist 300)
- 2 Luer 60 cc syringes (for contrast)
- 18 gauge needle (for drawing contrast)
- 19–21 gauge butterfly needle or angiocath
- Tourniquet
- Alcohol swab
- Tape (to secure IV)
- Small bandage

SCOUT FILM

- AP KUB
- Obliques (LPO/RPO) if suspicious calcifications are seen

SAMPLE DICTATION

The scout film reveals no suspicious calcifications or other significant abnormalities. After informed consent was obtained, 100 cc Oxilan 300 was administered through an antecubital vein. The immediate nephrogram showed equal opacification of both kidneys, which are normal in size, shape, and position. Excretion of contrast into the collecting systems was normal and equal at 5 minutes. The collecting systems appear normal, without filling defects or displacement. The ureters were fully opacified and are normal in course and caliber. There was no significant postvoid retention of contrast. ■

RADIATION

- Fluoro: 400 mrad/min
- Spot films: 40 mrad per spot film

EXAM

1 *Obtain Informed Consent*

Ask the patient about previous contrast reactions and location of pain, and obtain written consent if necessary. Verify that the patient does not have impaired renal function. Some institutions require serum BUN/creatinine measurements on all patients within 4 weeks. Explain the possible side effects of intravenous contrast material.

2 *Inspect Scout Film for Calculi*

Carefully inspect the scout film for suspicious calcifications. If calcifications project over the renal shadows, obtain oblique views for localization before injecting contrast into the patient.

TABLETOP
Horizontal

PATIENT
AP
±LPO/RPO

3 *Inject Contrast*

Start an antecubital vein IV and inject 100 cc contrast (50 cc if the patient has only one kidney), watching for extravasation. Leave the IV in place until the exam is complete.

TABLETOP
Head Up
30°

PATIENT
AP

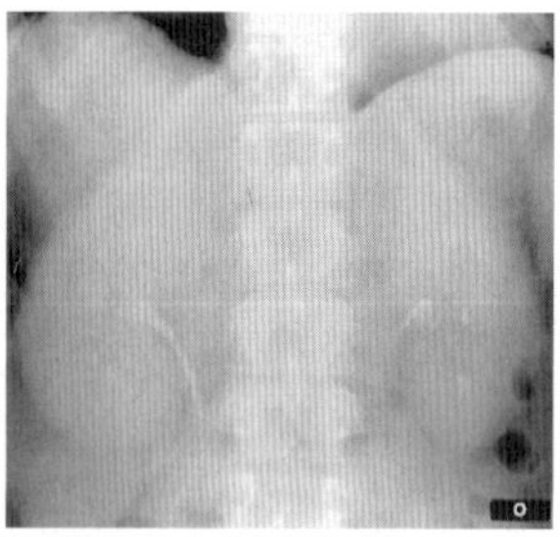

14 × 14
1 on 1

4 *Film Immediate Nephrogram*

Obtain the immediate nephrogram (this is considered the "0" minute nephrogram). Decline the tabletop −20° to promote filling of the collecting systems.

TABLETOP
Horizontal

75 kVp

PATIENT
AP

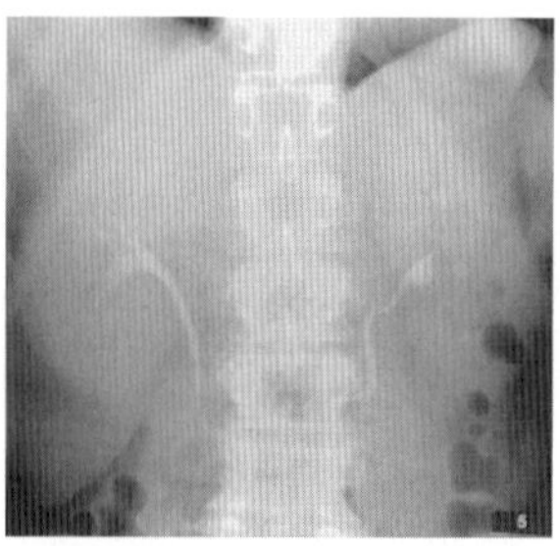

14 × 14
1 on 1

5 *Film 5 Minute Nephrogram*

After 5 minutes, image the kidneys and proximal ureters with a 14 × 14 cassette.

TABLETOP
Head Down
−20°

PATIENT
AP

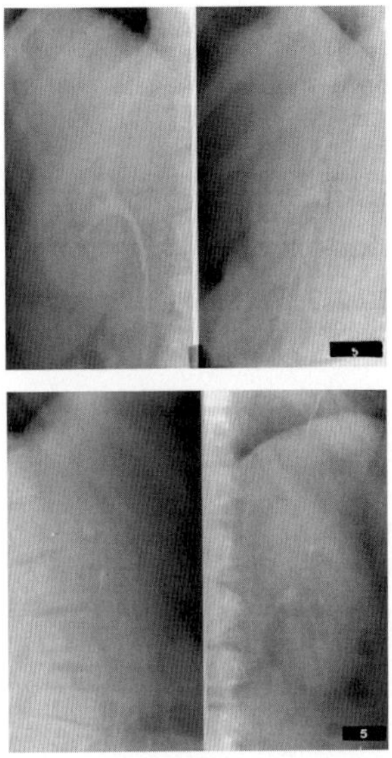

14 × 14
2 on 1
or
spot film

6 *Film Kidneys Individually*

Film each kidney in the following projections:

1. Right kidney (AP and RPO)
2. Left kidney (AP and LPO)

TABLETOP

Head Down

−20°

PATIENT

AP and RPO

AP and LPO

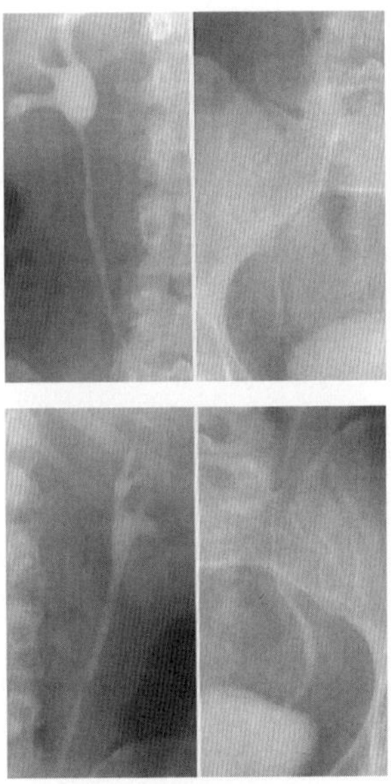

10 × 12
2 on 1
or
spot film
mag

7 *Film Ureters*

Elevate the tabletop to the horizontal position and film the ureters to (and including) the bladder. If the ureters are not visualized, raise the tabletop to 30–40°. This will cause the contrast that has accumulated in the renal collecting systems to be dumped into the ureters.

TABLETOP

Horizontal

PATIENT

AP

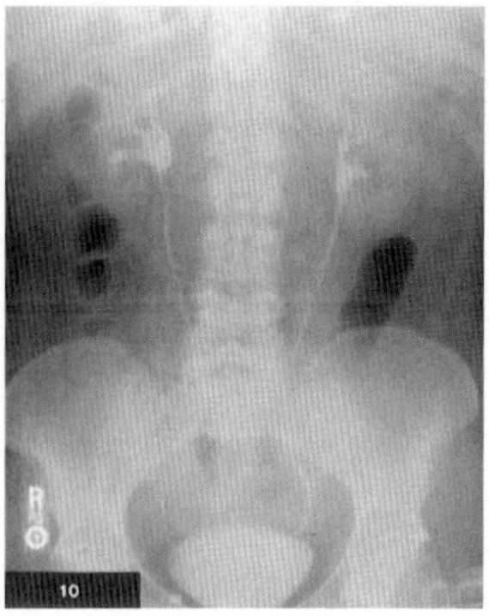

14 × 17

8 *Obtain Overhead Film*

At 10 minutes, have the technologist obtain an overhead KUB film. Send the patient to the restroom to void.

TABLETOP
Horizontal

75 kVp

PATIENT
AP

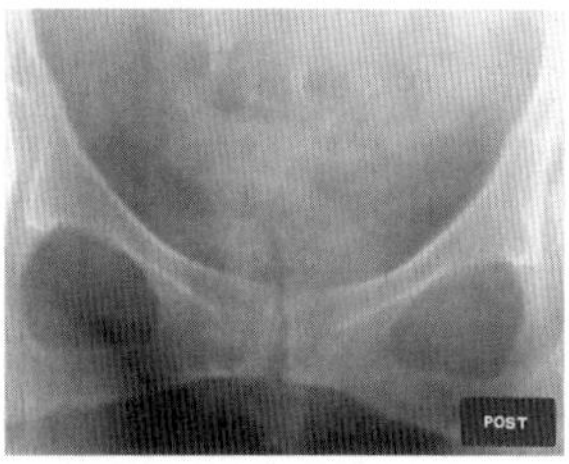

10 × 12
1 on 1
or
spot film

9 *Obtain Postvoid Film*

Obtain an AP postvoid film of the bladder. ■

TABLETOP
Horizontal

75 kVp

PATIENT
AP

Nephrostogram

INDICATIONS

- Evaluation for suspected urolithiasis
- Evaluation of collecting system/ureteral leakage
- Definition of collecting system/ureteral anatomy

CONTRAINDICATIONS

- No common contraindications

PATIENT PREPARATION

- None

SUPPLIES

- 50 cc 37% iodine water-soluble intravascular contrast (e.g., Hypaque-76, MD-76, RenoCal-76)
- 60 cc catheter tip or luer syringe (for contrast)
- 18 gauge needle (for drawing contrast)
- Alcohol swab
- 50 cc sterile saline
- 60 cc catheter tip or luer syringe (for saline)
- ±Plastic extension tubing

SCOUT FILM

- AP KUB

SAMPLE DICTATION

Approximately 40 cc RenoCal-76 was injected through the patient's existing right nephrostomy tube. Contrast opacified the dilated right renal collecting system and flowed freely through the entire right ureter and into the urinary bladder. Although there is residual dilatation of the proximal right ureter, no filling defects were identified. ■

RADIATION

- Fluoro: 400 mrad/min
- Spot films: 40 mrad per spot film

EXAM

1 *Prepare Contrast*

Choose an appropriate 60 cc syringe (e.g., catheter tip, luer) for the patient's nephrostomy tube and fill with contrast. Wipe the port of the nephrostomy tube with an alcohol swab. Connect the syringe to the nephrostomy tube and aspirate any air bubbles into the syringe.

If a C-arm fluoroscope is not being used, plastic extension tubing can be used to reach right-sided nephrostomy tubes.

TABLETOP
Horizontal

PATIENT
PA

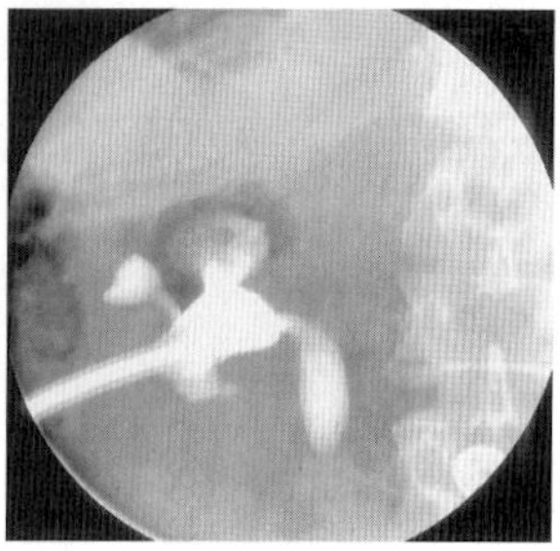

spot films
mag
or
14 × 14
2 on 1

2 *Image Collecting System*

Under fluoroscopic guidance, begin to inject contrast. Image the collecting system when it appears completely filled.

TABLETOP
Horizontal

75 kVp

PATIENT
PA

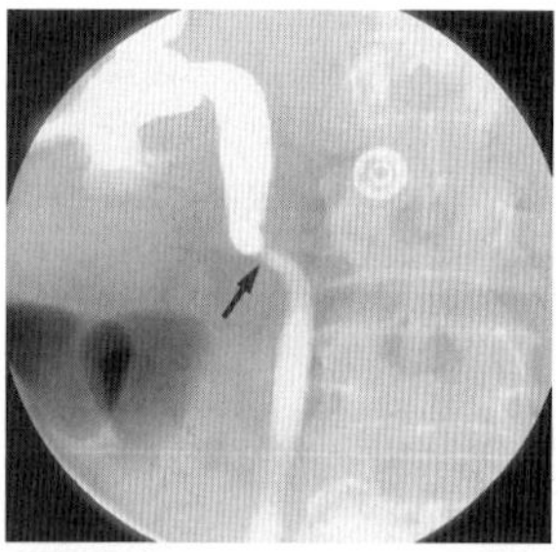

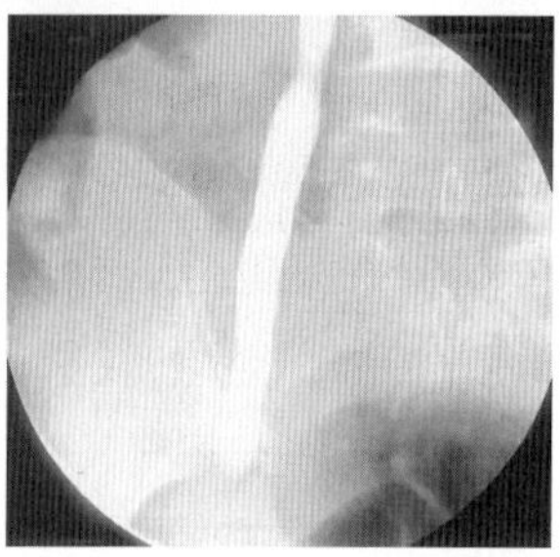

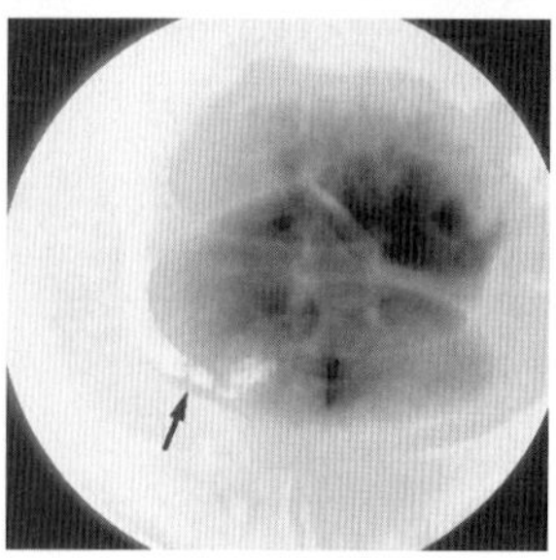

spot films
mag
or
14 × 14
2 on 1

3 *Image Ureter*

Continue injecting contrast to opacify the ureter. If an obstruction is encountered, obtain images for documentation; then wait a few minutes to observe for any contrast bypassing the obstruction.

If the nephrostomy tube is blocked and contrast is seen tracking back along the tube tract, obtain films for documentation.

Avoid overdistending the collecting system with contrast, which could result in rupture.

TABLETOP
Horizontal

PATIENT
PA

4 *Disconnect Tubing*

Have the films developed *before* removing the syringe. Flush the nephrostomy tube with sterile saline before reconnecting the drainage bag. ■

Hysterosalpingogram

INDICATIONS

- Infertility
- Delineation of uterine anatomy

CONTRAINDICATIONS

- Active pelvic inflammatory disease
- Perimenstrual period
- Recent conization, curettage, or pregnancy

PATIENT PREPARATION

- None

SUPPLIES

- 20 cc 37% iodine water-soluble intravascular contrast (e.g., Hypaque-76, MD-76, RenoCal-76)
- 20 cc control syringe (for contrast)
- 18 gauge needle (for drawing contrast)
- Plastic extension tubing
- Vaginal speculum
- Tenaculum
- Uterine sound
- 3 povidone-iodine swabs
- Lubrication jelly

SCOUT FILM

- AP pelvis

SAMPLE DICTATION

Approximately 7 cc RenoCal-76 was injected through the cervical canal, which was cannulated by the gynecologist. The endometrial cavity is normal in shape, size, and position. No intrauterine filling defects are present. There is synchronous filling of the fallopian tubes, with free spillage of contrast into the pelvic cavity. ■

RADIATION

- Fluoro: 500 mrad/min
- Spot films: 40 mrad per spot film

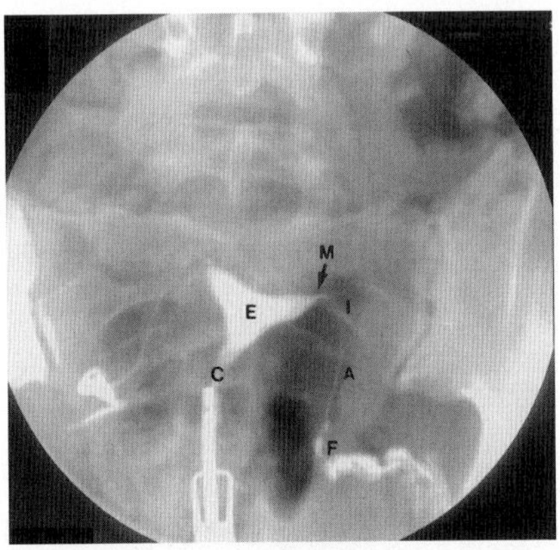

C—endocervical canal
E—endometrial cavity
M—intramural portion of fallopian tube
I—isthmus of fallopian tube
A—ampulla of fallopian tube
F—infundibulum of fallopian tube

FIGURE 1. *Uterine anatomy. Free spillage of contrast is present on the left. As spillage on the right may be contained, placing the patient in an oblique position is required to differentiate free and contained spillage.*

EXAM

1 Cannulate Cervical Canal

The patient is placed on the fluoroscopy table in the lithotomy position for cannulation of the cervical canal by the gynecologist.

When the gynecologist is ready for the injection, the patient is slowly moved toward the head of the table so that the pelvis can be imaged.

TABLETOP
Horizontal

PATIENT
Lithotomy

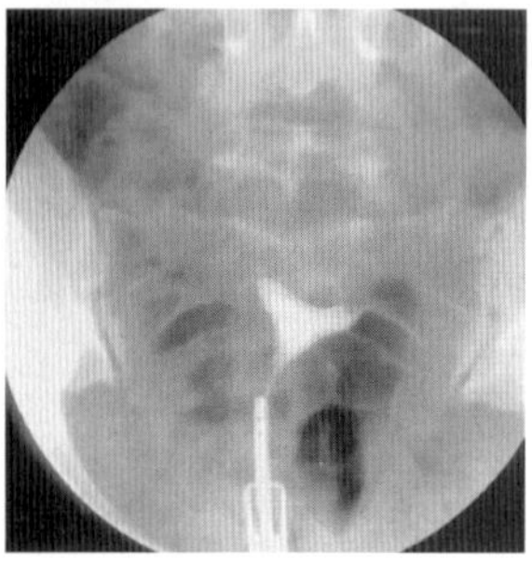

spot film
mag
or
10 × 12
2 on 1

2 Film Endometrial Cavity

Obtain sequential spot films as the gynecologist slowly injects contrast, showing filling of the endometrial cavity.

TABLETOP
Horizontal

75 kVp

PATIENT
AP

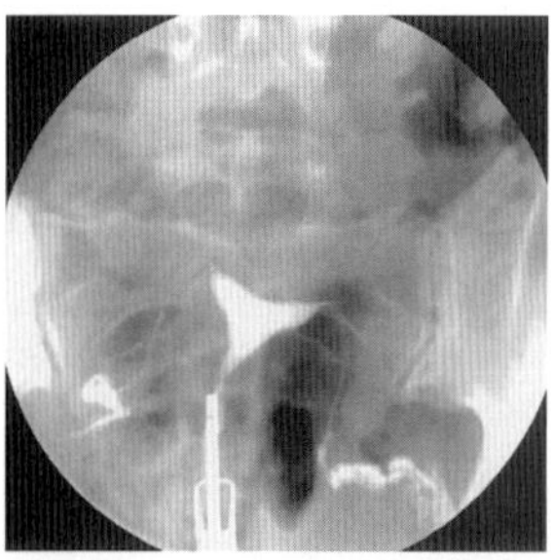

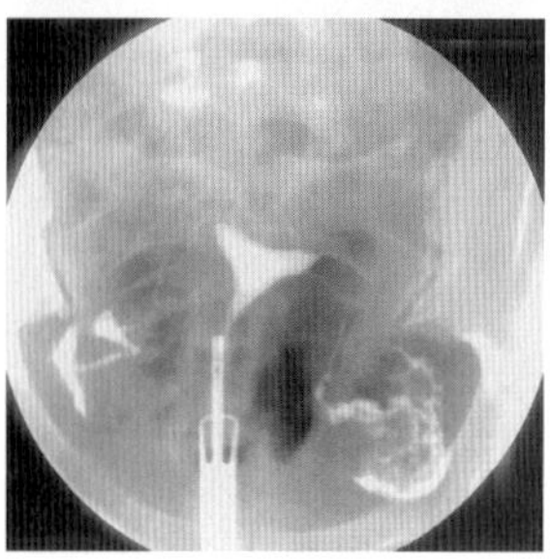

spot film
mag
or
10 × 12
1 on 1

3 Film Fallopian Tubes and Free Spillage

As more contrast is injected, obtain images demonstrating:

1. Filling of the fallopian tubes
2. Spillage into the pelvic cavity

If the filling of the fallopian tubes is asynchronous, it may be necessary to place the patient in an oblique position. This will isolate the spilled contrast away from the tube with delayed spillage so that contrast from the contralateral side is not mistaken for spillage from the other tube.

Make sure that free spillage is seen bilaterally. What may appear to be free spillage may actually be contained spillage. Free spillage can be assured if scalloping of the contrast is seen, representing contrast surrounding small bowel loops. ■

TABLETOP
Horizontal

PATIENT
AP
±RPO/LPO

PART VI

Musculoskeletal Examinations

Brock G. McDaniel, M.D.
Thomas P. Martin, M.D.

Shoulder Gadolinium Injection

Although commonly used for magnetic resonance arthrography, gadolinium has not yet been approved by the FDA for this purpose.

INDICATIONS

- Magnetic resonance imaging (MRI) evaluation of the rotator cuff and glenoid labrum with intra-articular gadolinium

CONTRAINDICATIONS

- Coagulopathy (relative)
- Soft tissue infection at puncture site
- Contrast allergy
- Contraindications to MRI, such as paramagnetic aneurysmal clips or cardiac pacemaker

PATIENT PREPARATION

- NPO 2 hours prior to exam

SUPPLIES

- Written consent form
- Metal hemostat
- Surgical marking pen
- Sterile gloves
- Povidone-iodine solution (e.g., Betadine)
- 3 prep swabs
- Sterile fenestrated drape
- Sterile 4 × 4 gauze
- Alcohol swab
- 5 cc 1% lidocaine without epinephrine
- 5 cc syringe (for lidocaine)
- 18 gauge needle (for drawing lidocaine and Gd/NaCl mixture)
- 1½ inch 25 gauge needle (for lidocaine)
- 0.3 cc gadolinium DTPA (e.g., Magnevist, Omniscan)
- Tuberculin syringe (for gadolinium)
- 50 cc bag normal saline
- 20 cc syringe (for Gd/NaCl mixture)
- 10 cc 20–30% iodine water-soluble contrast (e.g., Conray, Conray 43, Reno-60) (not sodium salt)
- 10 cc syringe (for iodinated contrast)
- Plastic extension tubing
- 20 gauge spinal needle with stylet (for joint injections)
- Antibiotic ointment
- Small bandage

SCOUT FILM

- Not obtained routinely
- Review prior radiographs

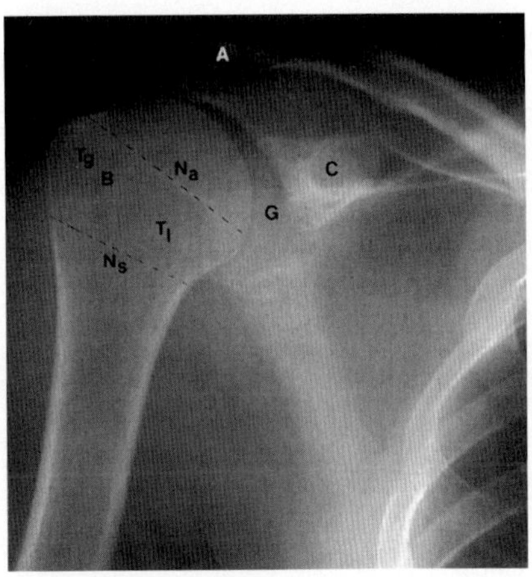

Tg—greater tubercle
Ti—lesser tubercle
C—coracoid
A—acromion
B—intubercular groove (bicipital groove)
Ns—surgical neck
Na—anatomic neck
G—glenoid

FIGURE 1. *Normal anatomy of the shoulder.*

SAMPLE DICTATION

Informed and written consent was obtained from the patient. The risks (including bleeding, infection, and capsular rupture), benefits, and alternatives to the exam were discussed. The patient was draped and prepared in a sterile fashion. The entrance site was localized using fluoroscopic guidance. Local anesthesia was achieved with 1% lidocaine solution. A 20 gauge spinal needle and stylet were introduced with fluoroscopic guidance into the right shoulder joint capsule, and approximately 2 cc Conray was instilled to confirm intra-articular positioning. Approximately 15 cc of a mixture of Magnevist and normal saline was instilled into the joint capsule. The needle was then removed, and the entrance site was dressed with antibiotic ointment and a bandage. There were no immediate postprocedure complications. ■

RADIATION

- Fluoro: 20 mrad/min
- Spot films: 10 mrad per spot film

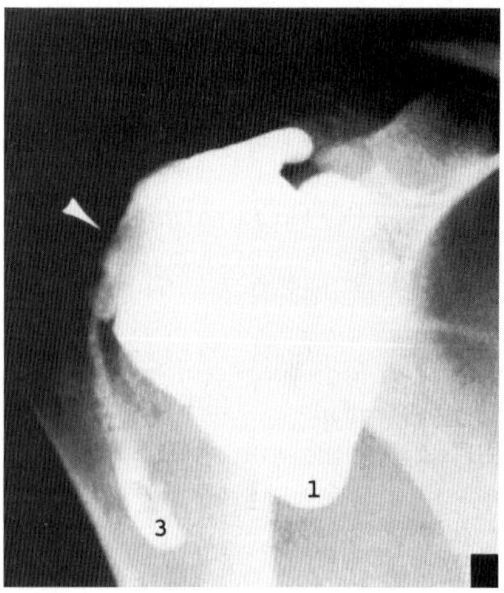

1—axillary pouch
3—bicipital tendon sheath
arrow—anatomic neck of the humerus

FIGURE 2. *Normal single contrast arthrogram of the shoulder (from Resnick D:* Bone and Joint Imaging, *2nd ed. Philadelphia, W.B. Saunders, 1996, p. 118).*

EXAM

1 *Obtain Informed Consent*

Obtain informed consent from the patient:

1. Risks: bleeding, infection, contrast reaction, joint capsule rupture
2. Benefits
3. Alternatives

Inform the patient about the signs and symptoms of infection (fever, pain and tenderness, swelling).

Verify that the MRI scanner will be available to image the patient after injection.

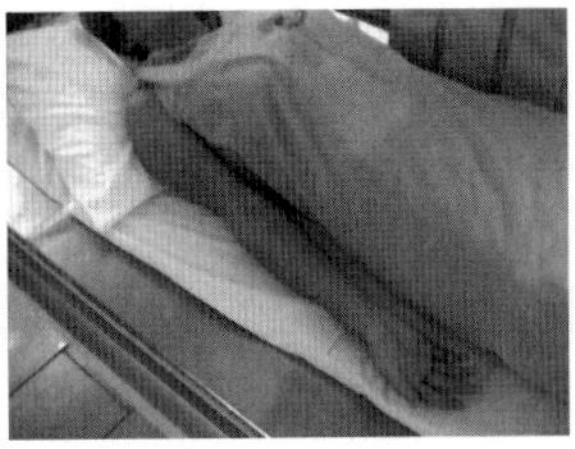

2 *Position Patient*

Have the patient lay supine on the fluoroscopy table with the hand supinated. Place a small sand bag or equivalent weight on the palm to stabilize this position. If a C-arm fluoroscope is not being used, position the patient's head at the foot of the table for a left shoulder arthrogram.

TABLETOP
Horizontal

PATIENT
AP

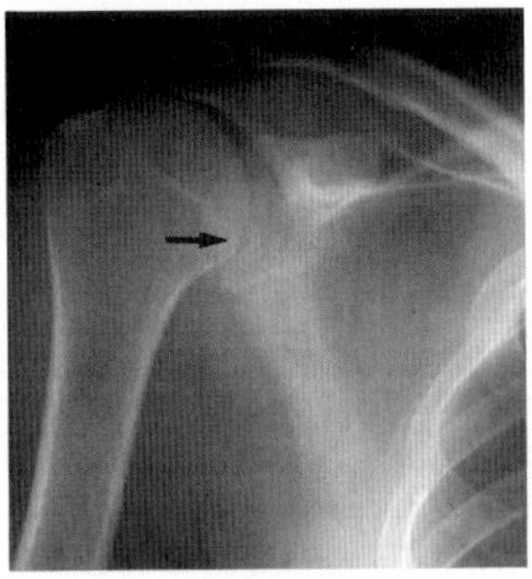

3 *Localize Entrance Site*

Using fluoroscopic guidance, locate the inferior aspect of the glenohumeral joint with a metal hemostat. Ensure that positioning is medial to the capsular attachment on the humeral head. Position the hemostat over the inferomedial humeral head, not directly over the joint, as the needle tends to be dragged medially. Mark this location by making a mark on the skin using a needle cap or a surgical marking pen.

TABLETOP
Horizontal

60 kVp

PATIENT
AP

℞

4 *Administer Local Anesthetic*

Using sterile technique, cleanse the overlying skin with povidone-iodine solution and apply the sterile fenestrated drape.

Anesthetize with 1% lidocaine along the anticipated needle course.

TABLETOP
Horizontal

PATIENT
AP

5 *Prepare Contrast Agents*

Draw 0.3 cc gadolinium into the tuberculin syringe. Add the gadolinium to the 50 cc bag of normal saline. Fill the 20 cc syringe with the Gd/NaCl mixture.

Fill the 10 cc syringe with the iodinated contrast; then attach it to the plastic extension tubing. Flush the tubing with contrast to expel all of the air from the system.

It is important to be meticulous about removing all of the air bubbles, because artifact from air injected into the joint will compromise the quality of the exam. Air bubbles mimic intra-articular loose bodies.

TABLETOP
Horizontal

PATIENT
AP

6 *Place Needle in Glenohumeral Joint*

Tent the skin over the insertion site. Direct the styletted 20 gauge spinal needle (bevel aiming laterally) into the joint space. Remember to position the needle over the inferomedial humeral head, not directly over the joint, as the needle tends to be dragged medially.

This should be a deliberate motion with minimal hesitation. If the needle is advanced too slowly, it tends to deflect and miss the desired target.

TABLETOP
Horizontal

PATIENT
AP

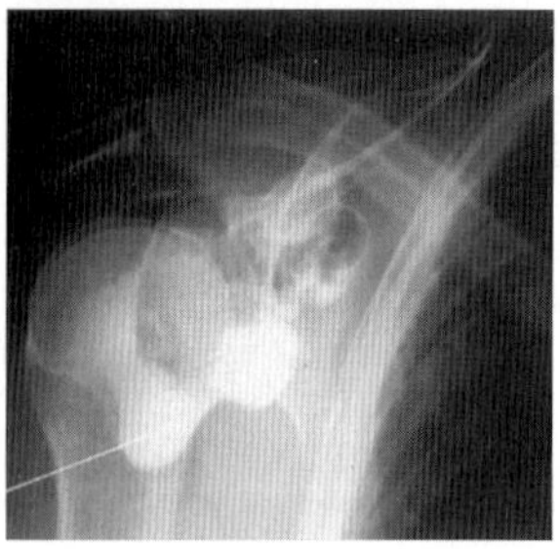

10 × 12
1 on 1
or
spot film

7 *Verify Proper Needle Placement*

Once the needle is felt to be inside the joint capsule, remove the stylet. Attach the extension tubing and syringe of iodinated contrast, being careful to remove any air bubbles. Using fluoroscopic guidance, inject a small amount of iodinated contrast into the joint capsule. Correct placement is assured when contrast is seen within the glenohumeral joint. Document intra-articular placement of contrast.

TABLETOP
Horizontal

PATIENT
AP

8 *Inject Gd/NaCl Mixture into Joint*

Attach the syringe containing the Gd/NaCl mixture to the extension tubing, being careful not to introduce any air bubbles into the tubing. Disconnect at the syringe hub, not the needle hub, allowing any residual contrast in the extension tubing to enter the joint upon injection. This ensures that the needle positioning is not disturbed. Inject 15–20 cc of the mixture into the joint space.

TABLETOP
Horizontal

PATIENT
AP

9 *Withdraw Needle*

Withdraw the spinal needle. Then clean the skin and cover the puncture site with antibiotic ointment and a small bandage.

TABLETOP
Horizontal

PATIENT
AP

10 *Obtain MRI*

Send the patient to the scanner for MRI imaging within a half hour of injecting the gadolinium contrast. ■

Elbow Gadolinium Injection

Although commonly used for magnetic resonance arthrography, gadolinium has not yet been approved by the FDA for this purpose.

INDICATIONS

- MRI evaluation of the elbow with intra-articular gadolinium

CONTRAINDICATIONS

- Coagulopathy (relative)
- Soft tissue infection at puncture site
- Contrast allergy
- Contraindications to MRI, such as paramagnetic aneurysmal clips or cardiac pacemaker

PATIENT PREPARATION

- NPO 2 hours prior to exam

SUPPLIES

- Written consent form
- Metal hemostat
- Surgical marking pen
- Sterile gloves
- Povidone-iodine solution (e.g., Betadine)
- 3 prep swabs
- Sterile fenestrated drape
- Sterile 4 × 4 gauze
- Alcohol swab
- 5 cc 1% lidocaine without epinephrine
- 5 cc syringe (for lidocaine)
- 18 gauge needle (for drawing lidocaine and Gd/NaCl mixture)
- 1½ inch 25 gauge needle (for lidocaine)
- 0.3 cc gadolinium DTPA (e.g., Magnevist, Omniscan)
- Tuberculin syringe (for gadolinium)
- 50 cc bag normal saline
- 20 cc syringe (for Gd/NaCl mixture)
- 10 cc 20–30% iodine water-soluble contrast (e.g., Conray, Conray 43, Reno-60) (not sodium salt)
- 10 cc syringe (for iodinated contrast)
- 1½ inch 22 gauge needle (for joint injections)
- Plastic extension tubing
- Antibiotic ointment
- Small bandage

SCOUT FILM

- Not obtained routinely
- Review prior radiographs

SAMPLE DICTATION

Informed and written consent was obtained from the patient. The risks (including bleeding, infection, and capsular rupture), benefits, and alternatives to the exam were discussed. The patient was draped and prepared in a sterile fashion. The entrance site was localized using fluoroscopic guidance. Local anesthesia was achieved with 1% lidocaine solu-

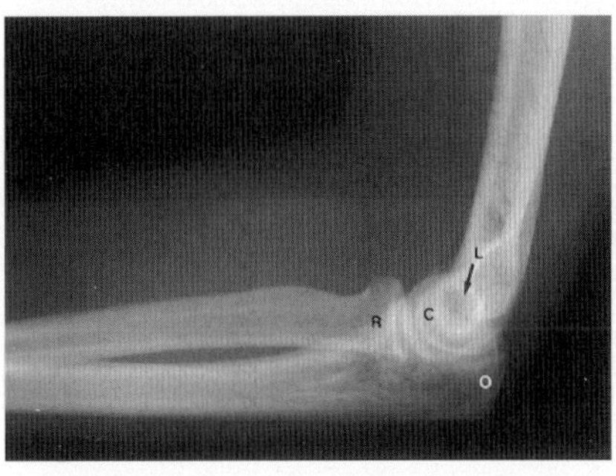

R—radial head
O—olecranon
C—capitulum
L—lateral epicondyle

FIGURE 1. *Normal anatomy of the elbow.*

tion. A 22 gauge needle was introduced with fluoroscopic guidance into the right radio-capitellar joint, and approximately 2 cc Conray was instilled to confirm intra-articular positioning. Approximately 9 cc of a mixture of Magnevist and normal saline was instilled into the joint capsule. The needle was then removed, and the entrance site was dressed with antibiotic ointment and a bandage. There were no immediate postprocedure complications. ■

RADIATION

- Fluoro: 10 mrad/min
- Spot films: 5 mrad per spot film

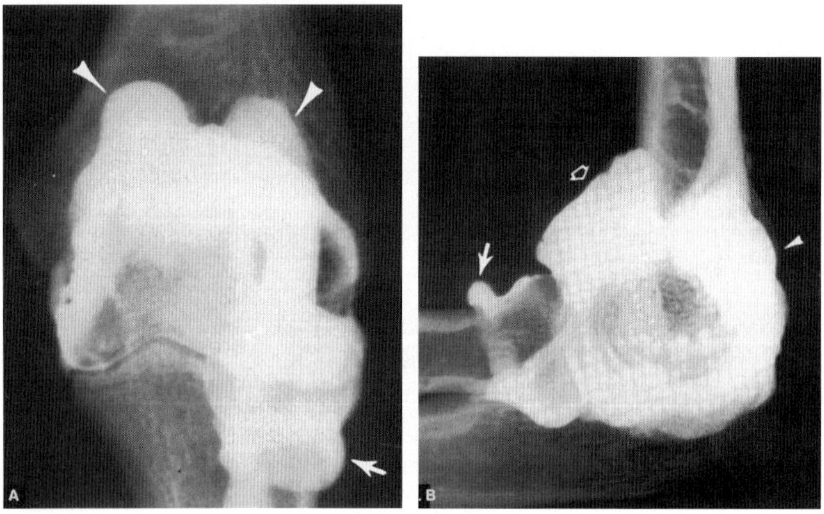

arrowheads (A)—Proximal extension of contrast in front of humerus

arrowhead (B)—olecranon (posterior) recess

arrows—periradial or annular recess

open arrow—coronoid (anterior) recess

FIGURE 2. *Normal arthrogram of the elbow in AP (A) and lateral (B) projections (from Resnick D:* Bone and Joint Imaging, *2nd ed. Philadelphia, W.B. Saunders, 1996, p. 116).*

EXAM

1 *Obtain Informed Consent*

Obtain informed consent from the patient:

1. Risks: bleeding, infection, contrast reaction, joint capsule rupture
2. Benefits
3. Alternatives

Inform the patient about the signs and symptoms of infection (fever, pain and tenderness, swelling).

Verify that the MRI scanner will be available to image the patient after injection.

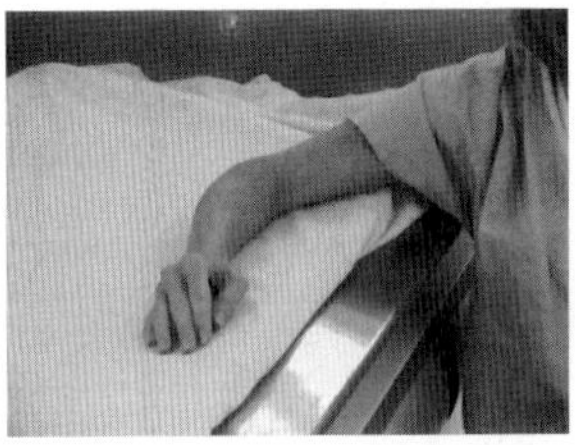

2 *Position Patient*

Have the patient wear a lead apron and sit on a stool next to the fluoroscopy table, with the elbow to be injected on the tabletop.

TABLETOP
Horizontal

PATIENT
Sitting

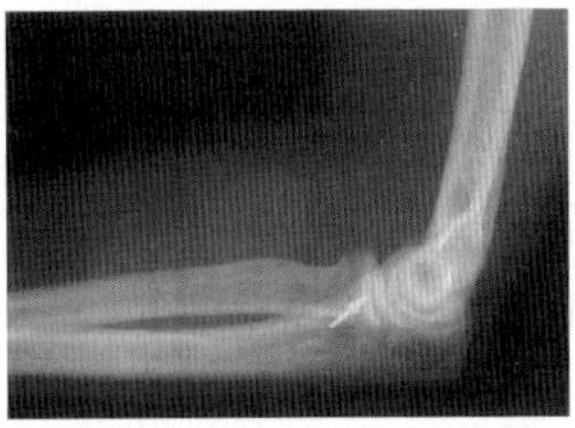

3 *Localize Entrance Site*

While palpating over the radial head, pronate the forearm and locate the joint space between the radial head and capitellum. Using fluoroscopic guidance, locate the radiocapitellar joint with a metal hemostat. Mark this location by making a mark on the skin using a needle cap or a surgical marking pen.

TABLETOP
Horizontal

60 kVp

PATIENT
Sitting

℞

4 *Administer Local Anesthetic*

Using sterile technique, cleanse the overlying skin with povidone-iodine solution and apply the sterile fenestrated drape.

Anesthetize with 1% lidocaine along the anticipated needle course.

TABLETOP
Horizontal

PATIENT
Sitting

5 *Prepare Contrast Agents*

Draw 0.3 cc gadolinium into the tuberculin syringe. Add the gadolinium to the 50 cc bag of normal saline. Fill the 20 cc syringe with the Gd/NaCl mixture.

Fill the 10 cc syringe with the iodinated contrast; then attach it to the plastic extension tubing. Flush the tubing with contrast to expel all of the air from the system.

It is important to be meticulous about removing all of the air bubbles because artifact from the air injected into the joint will compromise the quality of the exam. Air bubbles mimic intra-articular loose bodies.

TABLETOP
Horizontal

PATIENT
Sitting

6 *Place Needle in Radiocapitellar Joint*

Tent the skin over the insertion site. Using fluoroscopic guidance, direct the 1½ inch, 22 gauge needle into the joint space.

TABLETOP
Horizontal

PATIENT
Sitting

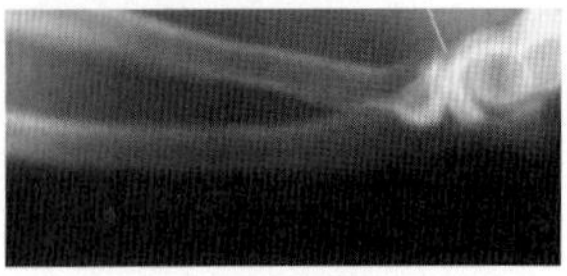

10 × 12
1 on 1
or
spot film

7 *Verify Proper Needle Placement*

Once the needle is felt to be inside the joint capsule, attach the extension tubing, being careful to remove any air bubbles. Using fluoroscopic guidance, inject a small amount of iodinated contrast into the joint capsule. Correct placement is assured when contrast is seen surrounding the capitellum. Document intra-articular placement of contrast.

TABLETOP
Horizontal

PATIENT
Sitting

8 *Inject Gd/NaCl Mixture into Joint*

Attach the syringe containing the Gd/NaCl mixture to the extension tubing, being careful not to introduce any air bubbles into the tubing. Disconnect at the tube hub, not the needle hub, allowing any residual contrast in the tubing to enter the joint upon injection. This ensures that the needle positioning is not disturbed. Inject 8–10 cc of the mixture into the joint space.

TABLETOP
Horizontal

PATIENT
Sitting

9 *Withdraw Needle*

Carefully withdraw the needle. Then clean the skin and cover the puncture site with antibiotic ointment and a small bandage.

TABLETOP
Horizontal

PATIENT
Sitting

10 *Obtain MRI*

Send the patient to the scanner for MRI imaging within a half hour of injecting the gadolinium contrast. ■

Wrist Gadolinium Injection

Although commonly used for magnetic resonance arthrography, gadolinium has not yet been approved by the FDA for this purpose.

INDICATIONS

- MRI evaluation for triangular fibrocartilage complex tear or ligamentous injury (i.e., scapholunate) with intra-articular gadolinium

CONTRAINDICATIONS

- Coagulopathy (relative)
- Soft tissue infection at puncture site
- Contrast allergy
- Contraindications to MRI, such as paramagnetic aneurysmal clips or cardiac pacemaker

PATIENT PREPARATION

- NPO 2 hours prior to exam

SUPPLIES

- Written consent form
- Metal hemostat
- Surgical marking pen
- Sterile gloves
- Povidone-iodine solution (e.g., Betadine)
- 3 prep swabs
- Sterile fenestrated drape
- Sterile 4 × 4 gauze
- Alcohol swab
- 5 cc 1% lidocaine without epinephrine
- 5 cc syringe (for lidocaine)
- 18 gauge needle (for drawing lidocaine and Gd/NaCl mixture)
- 1½ inch 25 gauge needle (for lidocaine and joint injections)
- 0.3 cc gadolinium DTPA (e.g., Magnevist, Omniscan)
- Tuberculin syringe (for gadolinium)
- 50 cc bag normal saline
- 10 cc syringe (for Gd/NaCl mixture)
- 10 cc 20–30% iodine water-soluble contrast (e.g., Conray, Conray 43, Reno-60) (not sodium salt)
- 10 cc syringe (for iodinated contrast)
- Plastic extension tubing
- Antibiotic ointment
- Small bandage

SCOUT FILM

- Not obtained routinely
- Review prior radiographs

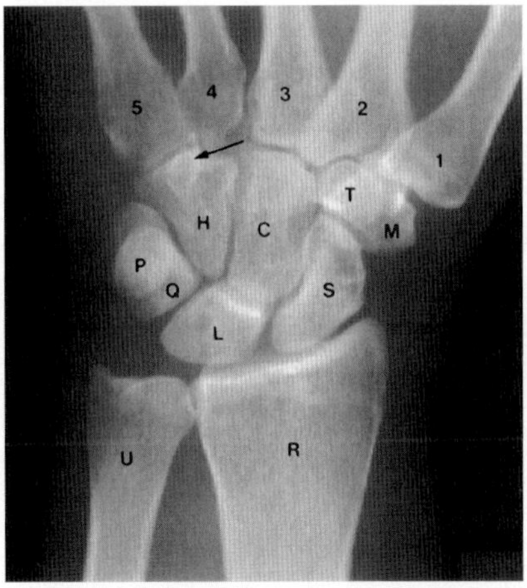

H—hamate
C—capitate
M—trapezium
T—trapezoid
P—pisiform
Q—triquetral
L—lunate
S—scaphoid
arrow—hook of hamate
U—ulna
R—radius
1–5—metacarpals

FIGURE 1. *Normal anatomy of the wrist.*

SAMPLE DICTATION

Informed and written consent was obtained from the patient. The risks (including bleeding, infection, and capsular rupture), benefits, and alternatives to the exam were discussed. The patient was draped and prepared in a sterile fashion. The entrance site was localized using fluoroscopic guidance. Local anesthesia was achieved with 1% lidocaine solution. A 25 gauge needle was introduced with fluoroscopic guidance into the right radioscaphoid joint, and approximately 1 cc Conray was instilled to confirm intra-articular positioning. Approximately 3 cc of a mixture of Magnevist and normal saline was instilled into the joint capsule. The needle was then removed, and the entrance site was dressed with antibiotic ointment and a bandage. There were no immediate postprocedure complications. ■

RADIATION

- Fluoro: 10 mrad/min
- Spot films: 5 mrad per spot film

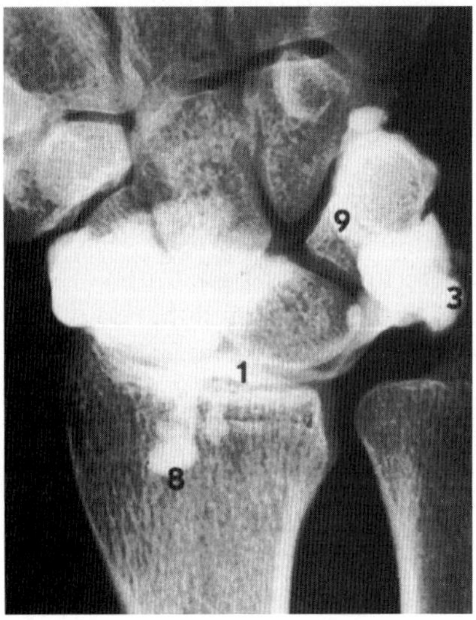

1—Radiocarpal compartment
3—Prestyloid recess
8—Volar radial recess
9—Pisiform triquetral compartment

FIGURE 2. *Normal arthrogram of the wrist (from Resnick D:* Bone and Joint Imaging, *2nd ed. Philadelphia, W.B. Saunders, 1996, p. 114).*

EXAM

1 *Obtain Informed Consent*

Obtain informed consent from the patient:

1. Risks: bleeding, infection, contrast reaction, joint capsule rupture
2. Benefits
3. Alternatives

TABLETOP

Horizontal

PATIENT

Sitting

1 *Obtain Informed Consent* *(continued)*

Inform the patient about the signs and symptoms of infection (fever, pain and tenderness, swelling). Some patients, especially younger ones, have a high incidence of vasovagal reactions to this procedure.

Verify that the MRI scanner will be available to image the patient after injection.

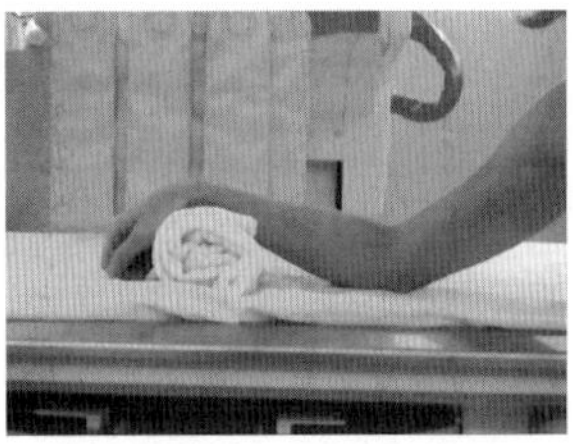

2 *Position Patient*

Have the patient wear a lead apron and sit on a stool next to the fluoroscopy table, with the wrist to be injected on the tabletop. Place a small foam wedge or rolled towel under the pronated wrist to achieve volar flexion.

TABLETOP
Horizontal

PATIENT
Sitting

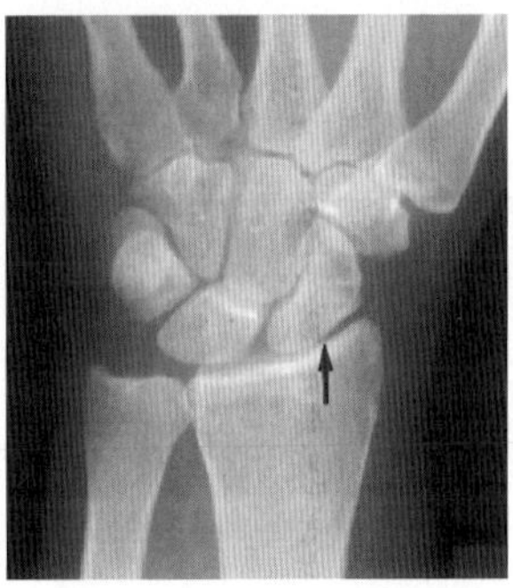

3 *Localize Entrance Site*

Using fluoroscopic guidance, locate the radioscaphoid joint. Position the hemostat over the joint, away from the scapholunate joint. Mark this location by making a mark on the skin using a needle cap or a surgical marking pen.

TABLETOP
Horizontal

55 kVp

PATIENT
Sitting

℞

4 *Administer Local Anesthetic*

Using sterile technique, cleanse the overlying skin with povidone-iodine solution and apply the sterile fenestrated drape.

Anesthetize the skin overlying the anticipated needle course with 1% lidocaine.

TABLETOP
Horizontal

PATIENT
Sitting

5 *Prepare Contrast Agents*

Draw 0.3 cc gadolinium into the tuberculin syringe. Add the gadolinium to the 50 cc bag of normal saline. Fill the 10 cc syringe with the Gd/NaCl mixture.

Fill the 10 cc syringe with the iodinated contrast; then attach it to the plastic extension tubing. Flush the tubing with contrast to expel all of the air from the system.

It is important to be meticulous about removing all of the air bubbles because artifact from the air injected into the joint will compromise the quality of the exam. Air bubbles mimic intra-articular loose bodies.

TABLETOP
Horizontal

PATIENT
Sitting

6 *Place Needle in Radioscaphoid Joint*

Tent the skin over the insertion site. Using fluoroscopic guidance, direct a 25 gauge needle into the joint space while injecting 1% lidocaine. A pop should be felt as the dorsal capsule is entered.

TABLETOP
Horizontal

PATIENT
Sitting

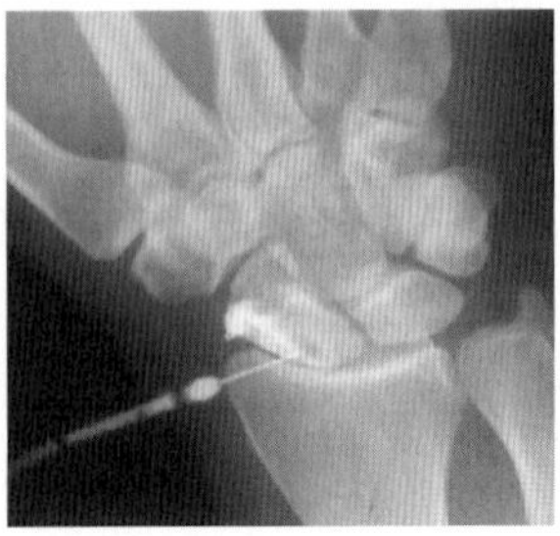

10 × 12
1 on 1
or
spot film

7 *Verify Proper Needle Placement*

Once the needle is felt to be inside the joint capsule, remove the syringe from the needle. Attach the extension tubing and iodinated contrast to the needle, being careful to remove any air bubbles. Using fluoroscopic guidance, inject a small amount of iodinated contrast into the joint capsule. Correct placement is assured when contrast is seen within the radioscaphoid joint. Document intra-articular placement of contrast.

TABLETOP
Horizontal

PATIENT
Sitting

8 *Inject Gd/NaCl Mixture into Joint*

Disconnect the extension tubing from the needle at the needle hub, not the syringe hub. Attach the syringe containing the Gd/NaCl mixture to the extension tubing and flush the tubing to expel all of the air from the system. Carefully attach the extension tubing to the needle and inject 3–4 cc of the Gd/NaCl mixture into the joint space.

TABLETOP
Horizontal

PATIENT
Sitting

9 *Withdraw Needle*

Carefully withdraw the needle. Then clean the skin and cover the puncture site with antibiotic ointment and a small bandage.

TABLETOP
Horizontal

PATIENT
Sitting

10 *Obtain MRI*

Send the patient to the scanner for MRI imaging immediately after injecting the gadolinium contrast. ■

Knee Gadolinium Injection

Although commonly used for magnetic resonance arthrography, gadolinium has not yet been approved by the FDA for this purpose.

INDICATIONS

- MRI evaluation of the knee with intraarticular gadolinium

CONTRAINDICATIONS

- Coagulopathy (relative)
- Soft tissue infection at puncture site
- Contrast allergy
- Contraindications to MRI, such as paramagnetic aneurysmal clips or cardiac pacemaker

PATIENT PREPARATION

- NPO 2 hours prior to exam

SUPPLIES

- Written consent form
- Surgical marking pen
- Sterile gloves
- Povidone-iodine solution (e.g., Betadine)
- 3 prep swabs
- Sterile fenestrated drape
- Sterile 4 × 4 gauze
- Alcohol swab
- 5 cc 1% lidocaine without epinephrine
- 5 cc syringe (for lidocaine)
- 18 gauge needle (for drawing lidocaine and Gd/NaCl mixture)
- 1½ inch 25 gauge needle (for lidocaine injection)
- 0.6 cc gadolinium DTPA (e.g., Magnevist, Omniscan)
- Tuberculin syringe (for gadolinium)
- 100 cc bag normal saline
- 60 cc syringe (for Gd/NaCl mixture)
- 10 cc 20–30% iodine water-soluble contrast (e.g., Conray, Conray 43, Reno-60) (not sodium salt)
- 10 cc syringe (for iodinated contrast)
- Plastic extension tubing
- 1½ inch 22 gauge needle (for joint injections)
- Antibiotic ointment
- Small bandage

SCOUT FILM

- Not obtained routinely
- Review prior radiographs

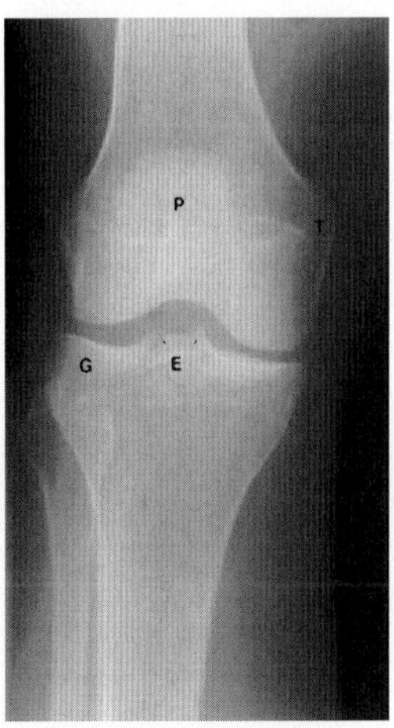

E—intercondylar eminence

G—Gerdy's tubercle (insertion of the iliotibial band)

P—patella

T—adductor tubercle

FIGURE 1. *Normal anatomy of the knee.*

SAMPLE DICTATION

Informed and written consent was obtained from the patient. The risks (including bleeding, infection, and capsular rupture), benefits, and alternatives to the exam were discussed. The patient was draped and prepared in a sterile fashion. The entrance site was localized using fluoroscopic guidance. Local anesthesia was achieved with 1% lidocaine solution. A 22 gauge needle was introduced with fluoroscopic guidance into the right patellofemoral joint, and approximately 6 cc Conray was instilled to confirm intra-articular positioning. Approximately 55 cc of a mixture of Magnevist and normal saline was instilled into the joint capsule. The needle was then removed, and the entrance site was dressed with antibiotic ointment and a bandage. There were no immediate postprocedure complications. ■

RADIATION

- Fluoro: 10 mrad/min
- Spot films: 5 mrad per spot film

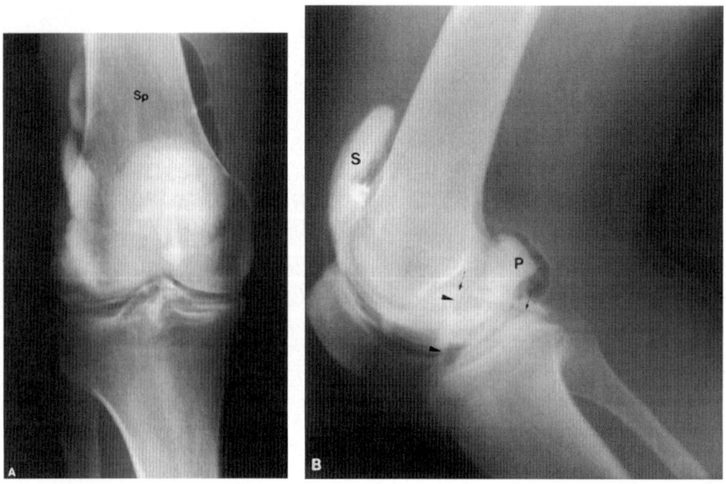

Sp—AP projection of the suprapatellar pouch
S—suprapatellar pouch
P—posterior extent of capsule
arrowheads—anterior cruciate ligament
arrow—posterior cruciate ligament

FIGURE 2. *Normal arthrogram of the knee in AP (A) and lateral (B) projections.*

EXAM

1 *Obtain Informed Consent*

Obtain informed consent from the patient:

1. Risks: bleeding, infection, contrast reaction, joint capsule rupture
2. Benefits
3. Alternatives

Inform the patient about the signs and symptoms of infection (fever, pain and tenderness, swelling).

Verify that the MRI scanner will be available to image the patient after injection.

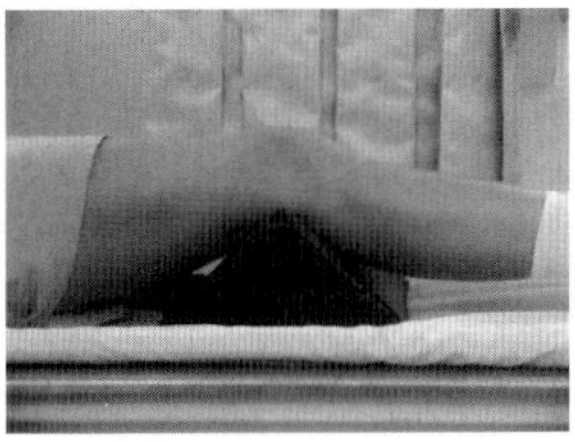

2 *Position Patient*

Have the patient lay supine on the fluoroscopy table with the knee slightly flexed. Place a small foam wedge under the knee. If a C-arm fluoroscope is not being used, position the patient's head at the foot of the table for a left knee arthrogram.

TABLETOP
Horizontal

PATIENT
AP

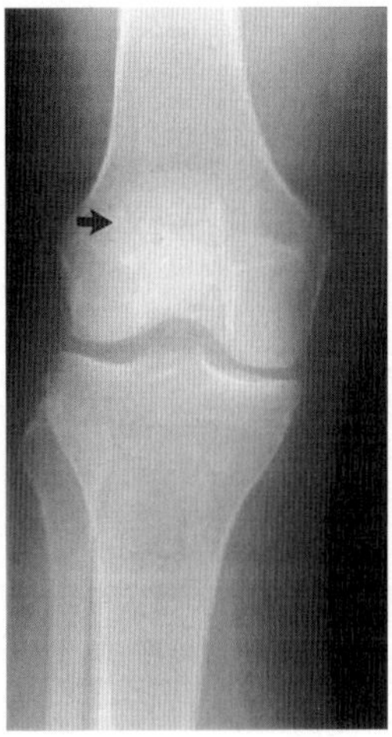

3 *Localize Entrance Site*

Locate the inferior aspect of the patella by palpation. Have the patient completely relax the knee. The joint will be entered along the lateral aspect of the patellofemoral compartment. Mark this location by making a mark on the skin using a needle cap or a surgical marking pen.

TABLETOP
Horizontal

60 kVp

PATIENT
AP

℞

4 *Administer Local Anesthetic*

Cleanse the overlying skin with povidone-iodine solution and apply the sterile fenestrated drape. Wipe the anticipated puncture site with an alcohol swab.

Anesthetize with 1% lidocaine along the anticipated needle course.

TABLETOP
Horizontal

PATIENT
AP

5 *Prepare Contrast Agents*

Draw 0.6 cc gadolinium into the tuberculin syringe. Add the gadolinium to the 100 cc bag of normal saline. Fill the 60 cc syringe with the Gd/NaCl mixture.

Fill the 10 cc syringe with the iodinated contrast; then attach it to the plastic extension tubing. Flush the tubing with contrast to expel all of the air from the system.

It is important to be meticulous about removing all of the air bubbles because artifact from the air injected into the joint will compromise the quality of the exam. Air bubbles mimic intra-articular loose bodies.

TABLETOP
Horizontal

PATIENT
AP

6 *Place Needle in Patellofemoral Joint*

Instruct the patient to relax the knee. Depress the medial aspect of the patella while displacing the patella laterally to open the lateral joint space. Using the thumb of the same hand, palpate the lateral articular surface of the patella. From the lateral aspect of the joint, direct the 1½ inch 22 gauge needle medially so that it skims along the inferior aspect of the patella to enter the patellofemoral joint.

TABLETOP
Horizontal

PATIENT
AP

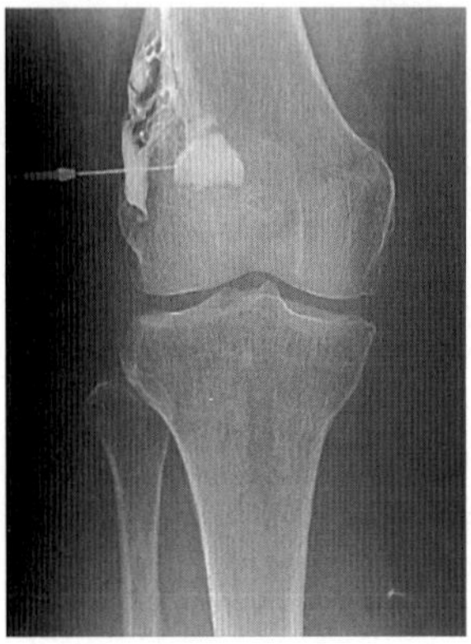

10 × 12
1 on 1
or
spot film

7 *Verify Proper Needle Placement*

Once the needle is felt to be inside the joint capsule, attach the extension tubing, being careful to remove any air bubbles. Using fluoroscopic guidance, inject a small amount of iodinated contrast into the joint capsule. Correct placement is assured when contrast is seen within the suprapatellar bursae. Document intra-articular placement of contrast.

TABLETOP
Horizontal

PATIENT
AP

8 *Inject Gd/NaCl Mixture into Joint*

Attach the syringe containing the Gd/NaCl mixture to the extension tubing, being careful not to introduce any air bubbles into the tubing. Disconnect at the tube hub, not the needle hub, allowing any residual contrast in the tubing to enter the joint upon injection. This ensures that the needle positioning was not disturbed. Inject 50–60 cc of the mixture into the joint space.

TABLETOP
Horizontal

PATIENT
AP

9 *Withdraw Needle*

Carefully withdraw the needle. Then clean the skin and cover the puncture site with antibiotic ointment and a small bandage.

TABLETOP
Horizontal

PATIENT
AP

10 *Obtain MRI*

Send the patient to the scanner in a wheelchair for MRI imaging within a half hour of injecting the gadolinium contrast. ■

Fluoroscopically Guided Hip Aspiration

INDICATIONS

- Suspected septic hip

CONTRAINDICATIONS

- Coagulopathy (relative)
- Soft tissue infection at puncture site

PATIENT PREPARATION

- NPO 2 hours prior to exam

SUPPLIES

- Written consent form
- Metal hemostat
- Surgical marking pen
- Sterile gloves
- Povidone-iodine solution (e.g., Betadine)
- 3 prep swabs
- Sterile fenestrated drape
- Sterile 4 × 4 gauze
- Alcohol swab
- 5 cc 1% lidocaine without epinephrine
- 5 cc syringe (for lidocaine)
- 18 gauge needle (for drawing lidocaine)
- 1 ½ inch 25 gauge needle (for lidocaine)
- 20 cc syringe (for joint aspiration)
- 10 cc 20–30% iodine water-soluble contrast (e.g., Conray, Conray 43, Reno-60) (not sodium salt)
- 10 cc syringe (for iodinated contrast)
- Plastic extension tubing
- 20 gauge spinal needle with stylet (for joint aspiration)
- 3 or 4 collection tubes
- Antibiotic ointment
- Small bandage

SCOUT FILM

- Not obtained routinely

SAMPLE DICTATION

Informed and written consent was obtained from the patient. The risks (including bleeding and infection), benefits, and alternatives to the exam were discussed. The patient was draped and prepared in a sterile fashion. The entrance site was localized utilizing fluoroscopic guidance. Local anesthesia was achieved with 1% lidocaine solution. A 20 gauge needle was introduced with fluoroscopic guidance into the right hip joint, and approximately 30 cc turbid fluid was aspirated. Approximately 6 cc Conray was instilled to confirm intra-articular positioning. The needle was then removed, and the en-

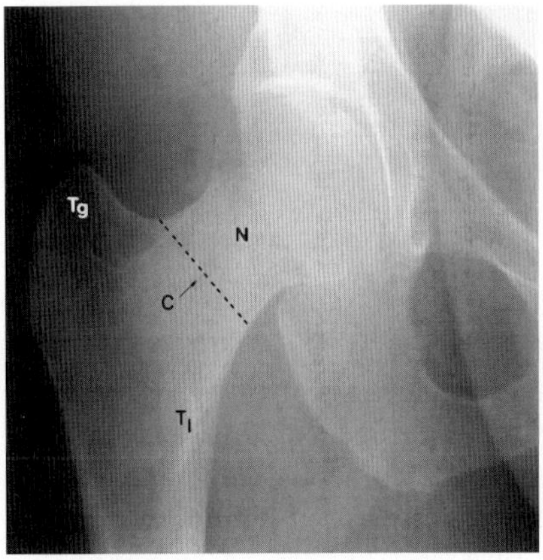

Tg—greater trochanter
Tl—lesser trochanter
C—line of capsular reflection
N—neck

FIGURE 1. *Normal anatomy of the hip.*

trance site was dressed with antibiotic ointment and a bandage. There were no immediate postprocedure complications. The aspirate was sent to the laboratory for Gram stain, culture, and sensitivity. ■

RADIATION

- Fluoro: 650 mrad/min
- Spot films: 40 mrad per spot film

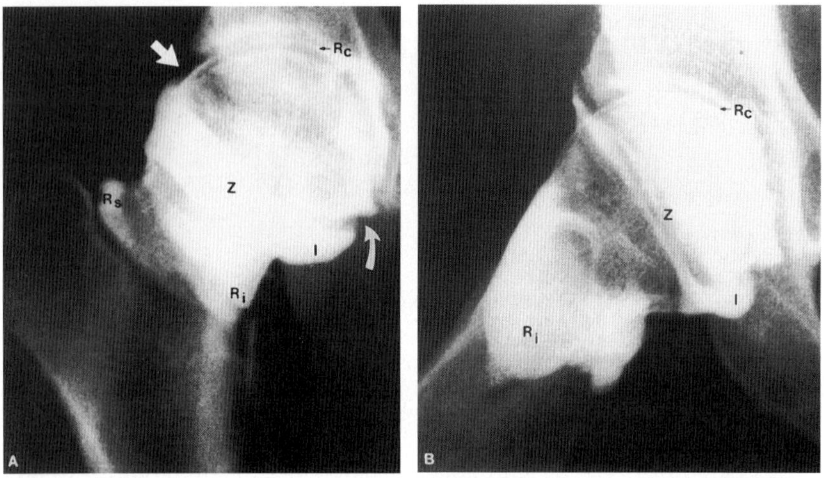

arrow—labrum
Z—zona orbicularis
curved arrow—ligamentum transversum
I—inferior articular recess
R_i—recess colli inferior
R_s—recess colli superior
R_c—recess capitus

FIGURE 2. *Normal arthrogram of the hip in AP (A) and lateral (B) projections (from Freiberger RH, Kaye JJ, Spiller J:* Arthrography. *Norwalk, CT, Appleton-Century-Crofts, 1979, p. 196; reprinted by permission of The McGraw-Hill Companies, Inc.).*

EXAM

1 *Obtain Informed Consent*

Obtain informed consent from the patient:

1. Risks: bleeding, infection, contrast reaction, joint capsule rupture
2. Benefits
3. Alternatives

Inform the patient about the signs and symptoms of infection (fever, pain and tenderness, swelling).

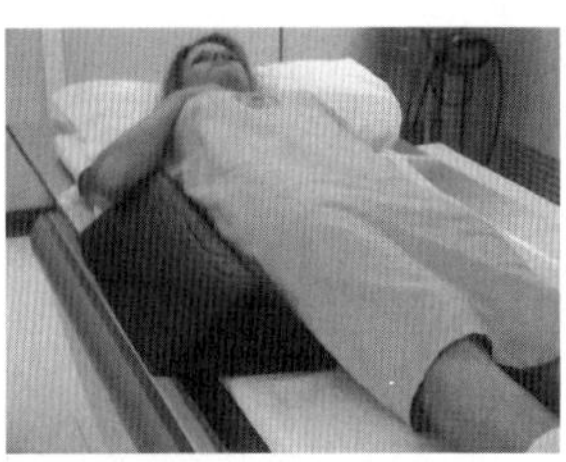

2 *Position Patient*

Palpate and localize the femoral artery. Have the patient lay supine on the fluoroscopy table, with the hip obliqued anteriorly 10° utilizing a foam wedge. If a C-arm fluoroscope is not being used, position the patient's head at the foot of the table for a left hip aspiration.

TABLETOP

Horizontal

PATIENT

LPO/RPO

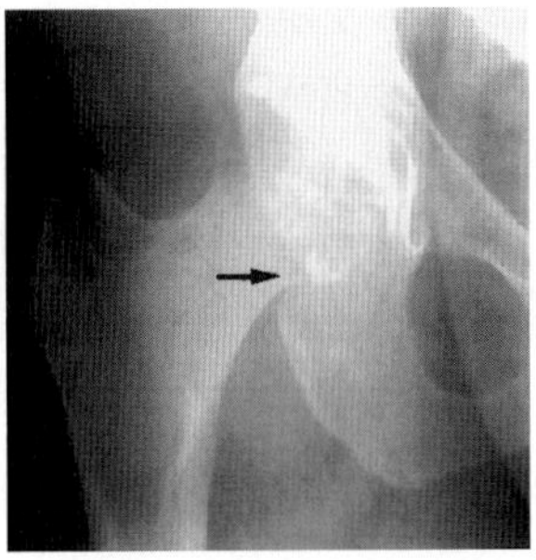

3 *Localize Entrance Site*

Using fluoroscopic guidance, locate the inferior aspect of the femoral head-neck junction with a metal hemostat. Ensure that positioning is medial to the capsular attachment and away from the femoral artery. Mark this location by making a mark on the skin using a needle cap or a surgical marking pen.

TABLETOP
Horizontal

70 kVp

PATIENT
LPO/RPO

℞

4 *Administer Local Anesthetic*

Cleanse the overlying skin with povidone-iodine solution and apply the sterile fenestrated drape.

Anesthetize with 1% lidocaine along the anticipated needle course.

TABLETOP
Horizontal

PATIENT
LPO/RPO

5 *Prepare Iodinated Contrast*

Fill the 10 cc syringe with the iodinated contrast; then attach it to the plastic extension tubing. Flush the tubing with contrast to expel all of the air from the system.

TABLETOP
Horizontal

PATIENT
LPO/RPO

6 *Place Needle in Hip Joint*

Tent the skin over the insertion site. Direct the styletted 20 gauge spinal needle (bevel aiming superiorly) into the joint space. Advance the needle until it impacts on the underlying femur. Retract the needle slightly so that the tip is in the joint capsule.

TABLETOP
Horizontal

PATIENT
LPO/RPO

7 *Aspirate Joint Fluid*

Once the needle is felt to be inside the joint capsule, remove the stylet from the spinal needle. Attach the 20 cc syringe to the spinal needle, being careful not to dislodge the needle.

Using the 20 cc syringe, attempt to aspirate fluid. If no fluid can be aspirated, flush the needle with preservative-free saline and reattempt to aspirate fluid. This process may need to be repeated several times to be successful.

Place the aspirated fluid in the collection tubes and send it to the laboratory for culture and sensitivity, Gram stain, and fungal culture (if indicated).

TABLETOP
Horizontal

PATIENT
LPO/RPO

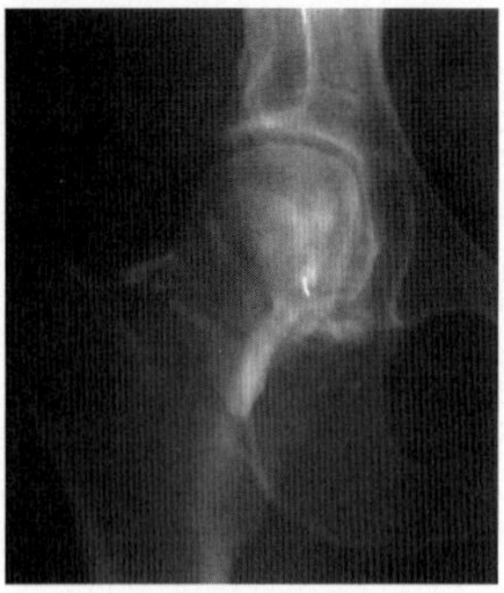

10 × 12
1 on 1
or
spot film

8 *Document Needle Placement*

Inject a small amount of iodinated contrast into the joint capsule. Correct placement is assured when contrast is seen within the hip joint. Document the needle placement.

TABLETOP
Horizontal

PATIENT
LPO/RPO

9 *Withdraw Needle*

Replace the stylet and carefully withdraw the spinal needle and stylet. Then clean the skin and cover the puncture site with antibiotic ointment and a small bandage. ■

TABLETOP
Horizontal

PATIENT
LPO/RPO

PART VII

Neuroradiology Examinations

Jeffrey D. Houston, M.D.
Frederick W. Rupp, M.D.

Fluoroscopically Guided Lumbar Puncture

INDICATIONS

- Unsuccessful blind lumbar puncture for cerebrospinal fluid collection

CONTRAINDICATIONS

- Increased intracranial pressure
- Soft tissue infection at puncture site
- Coagulopathy (relative contraindication)

PATIENT PREPARATION

- Historically, medications that lower seizure threshold (e.g., phenothiazines, antipsychotics, tricyclic antidepressants, central nervous system (CNS) stimulants, monoamine oxidase inhibitors, lithium, reserpine, isoniazid) have been discontinued 24–48 hours prior to nonemergent exams
- NPO after midnight or 6 hours prior to nonemergent exams

SUPPLIES

- Written consent form
- Metal hemostat
- Surgical marking pen
- Sterile gloves
- Povidone-iodine solution (e.g., Betadine)
- 3 prep swabs
- Alcohol swab
- Sterile 4 × 4 gauze
- Sterile fenestrated drape
- 5 cc 1% lidocaine without epinephrine
- 5 cc syringe (for lidocaine)
- 1½ inch 25 gauge needle (for lidocaine)
- 18 gauge needle (for drawing lidocaine)
- 3½ inch 22 gauge spinal needle with stylet
- ±Manometer
- ±Stopcock
- Short plastic extension tubing
- 3 or 4 numbered collection tubes (for concurrent cerebrospinal fluid collection)
- Antibiotic ointment
- Small bandage

SCOUT FILM

- PA lumbar spine

SAMPLE DICTATION

Informed and written consent was obtained from the patient. The risks (including bleeding, infection, and seizures), benefits, and alternatives to the exam were discussed. The patient was placed in the prone oblique position on the fluoroscopy table, and was prepared and draped in a sterile fashion. Local anesthesia was achieved using 1% lidocaine solution. The L2-L3 interspace was localized, and a 3½ inch 22 gauge spinal needle and stylet were advanced into the thecal sac under fluoroscopic guidance. Approximately 6 cc of clear cerebrospinal fluid was passively obtained and sent to the laboratory for Gram stain, culture, and sensitivity. The stylet was replaced, and the spinal needle was removed. There were no immediate postprocedure complications. ■

RADIATION

- Fluoro: 250 mrad/min
- Spot films: 50 mrad per spot film

EXAM

1 *Obtain Informed Consent*

Obtain informed consent from the patient or surrogate:

1. Risks: bleeding, infection, pain, headaches, seizures
2. Benefits
3. Alternatives

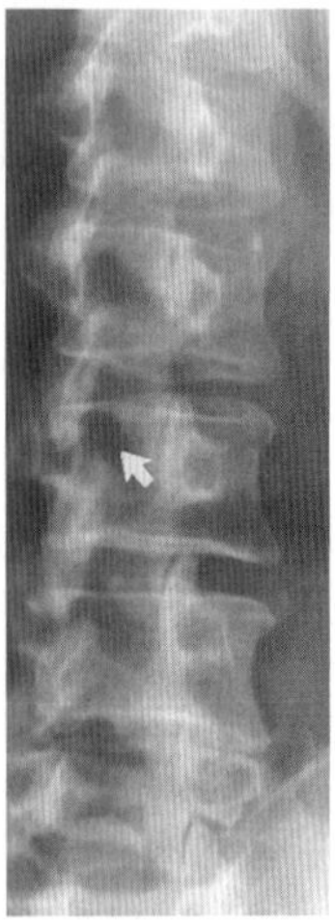

2 *Localize Access Site*

TABLETOP
Horizontal

75 kVp

PATIENT
LAO/RAO

Inspect the scout film for variant spinal anatomy and select the site of optimal access. Unless there is a contraindication, the L2-L3 interspace is often utilized because of an increased incidence of degenerative pathology at the lower lumbar levels. However, lumbar puncture at any lower lumbar level can be performed. Lumbar puncture should be avoided cephalad to L2 to prevent inadvertent injury to the cord.

Place the patient prone on the fluoroscopy table. Under fluoroscopic guidance, use a metal hemostat to localize the anticipated level of access. Slightly oblique the patient to allow visualization of a vertical course under the lamina into the thecal sac. Collimate as needed to focus on the spine.

Make a mark on the skin using a needle cap or a surgical marking pen at the site of anticipated puncture.

℞

3 *Administer Local Anesthetic*

TABLETOP
Horizontal

PATIENT
LAO/RAO

Using sterile technique, cleanse the overlying skin with povidone-iodine solution. Then wipe the anticipated puncture site with an alcohol swab.

Anesthetize with 1% lidocaine along the anticipated needle course.

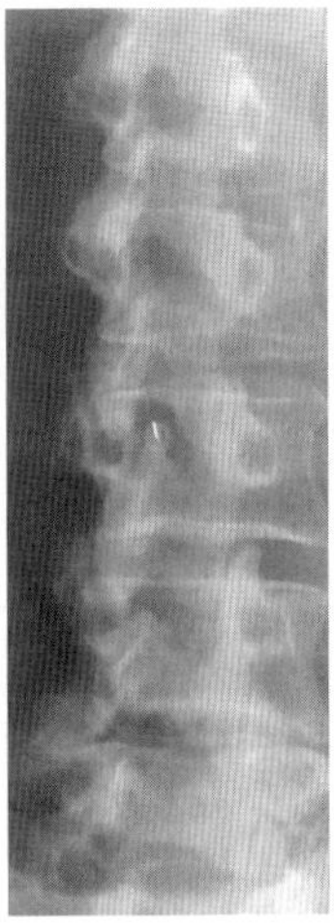

4 *Insert Spinal Needle*

Shallowly insert the spinal needle (with the stylet in place), keeping the notch on the needle hub directed perpendicular to the long axis of the spine so that the bevel of the needle will separate (not transect) the dural fibers.

The needle should be precisely positioned in both the horizontal and vertical axes so that it superimposes upon itself.

TABLETOP
Horizontal

PATIENT
LAO/RAO

5 *Access Thecal Sac*

Continue to advance the needle under intermittent fluoroscopic guidance into the soft tissues and verify that the needle is on course.

Elevate the patient's head to allow hydrostatic pressure to expand the thecal sac. Continue advancing the needle until the slight resistance of the ligamentum flavum is felt, followed by resistance of the dura, before entering the subarachnoid space. A second pop should be felt as the thecal sac is entered. The stylet should be periodically removed to check for the flow of cerebrospinal fluid. If there is no return of cerebrospinal fluid at the expected depth, a cross-table lateral film can be obtained to confirm correct needle placement.

TABLETOP
Head Up
15°

PATIENT
LAO/RAO

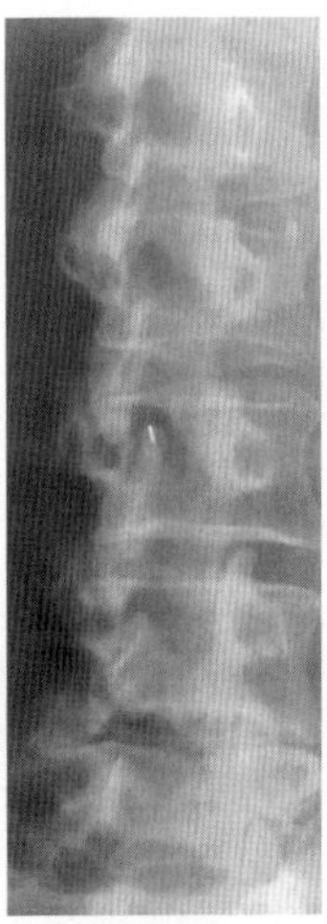

14 × 14
1 on 1
or
spot film

6 *Document Needle Placement*

Document the needle placement.

TABLETOP
Horizontal

PATIENT
LAO/RAO

7 *Perform Manometry*

If an opening pressure reading is desired, remove the stylet and carefully place the manometer (with or without a stopcock) into the spinal needle hub (with the table in a true horizontal position), open the stopcock (if used) to the manometer, and record the opening pressure in centimeters of water.

TABLETOP
Horizontal

PATIENT
LAO/RAO

8 *Collect Cerebrospinal Fluid*

Passively collect a sufficient quantity of cerebrospinal fluid, divided between three or four numbered collection tubes. The maximum amount of extracted fluid should generally not exceed 10–12 cc.

TABLETOP
Horizontal

PATIENT
LAO/RAO

9 *Withdraw Spinal Needle*

Replace the stylet and carefully withdraw the spinal needle and stylet. Then clean the skin and cover the puncture site with antibiotic ointment and a small bandage.

TABLETOP
Horizontal

PATIENT
LAO/RAO

10 *Write Postprocedure Orders*

The patient should be directed to restrict activity for 24 hours, to drink plenty of fluids, and to avoid bending or heavy lifting. Restricted medications can be resumed after 24 hours. ■

Lumbar Myelogram

Lumbar myelography is routinely performed with a combination of conventional imaging and computed tomography (CT) after intrathecal administration of iodinated contrast.

INDICATIONS

- Contraindication to MRI (e.g., pacemaker, aneurysm clip, claustrophobia, metal implants)
- Confirmation of equivocal MRI findings

CONTRAINDICATIONS

- Increased intracranial pressure
- Soft tissue infection at puncture site
- Coagulopathy (relative contraindication)
- Contrast allergy

PATIENT PREPARATION

- NPO after midnight or 6 hours prior to exam
- Historically, medications that lower seizure threshold (e.g., phenothiazines, antipsychotics, tricyclic antidepressants, CNS stimulants, monoamine oxidase inhibitors, lithium, reserpine, isoniazid) have been discontinued 24–48 hours prior to nonemergent exams.

SUPPLIES

- Written consent form
- Metal hemostat
- Surgical marking pen
- Sterile gloves
- Nonionic contrast approved for myelography (e.g., Omnipaque 180/240/300, Isovue-M 200/300)
- 20 cc syringe (for contrast)
- 18 gauge needle (for drawing contrast)
- Povidone-iodine solution (e.g., Betadine)
- 3 prep swabs
- Alcohol swab
- Sterile 4 × 4 gauze
- Sterile fenestrated drape
- 5 cc 1% lidocaine without epinephrine
- 5 cc syringe (for lidocaine)
- 1½ inch 25 gauge needle (for lidocaine)
- 18 gauge needle (for drawing lidocaine)
- 3½ inch 22 gauge spinal needle with stylet
- Long plastic extension tubing
- Antibiotic ointment
- Small bandage

SCOUT FILM

- Complete lumbar spine series

SAMPLE DICTATION

Informed and written consent was obtained from the patient. The risks (including bleeding, infection, and seizures), benefits, and alternatives to the exam were discussed. The patient was placed in the prone oblique position on the fluoroscopy table, and was prepared and draped in a sterile fashion. Local anesthesia was achieved using 1% lidocaine solution. The L2-L3 interspace was localized, and a 3½ inch 22 gauge spinal needle and stylet were advanced into the thecal sac under fluoroscopic guidance. Approximately 11 cc Isovue-M 200 was instilled into the thecal sac. The stylet was replaced, and the spinal needle was removed. Conventional lumbar myelogram films were then obtained. There is no evidence of lumbar nerve root compression, arachnoiditis, or extradural impression upon the thecal sac. There were no immediate postprocedure complications. ■

RADIATION

- Fluoro: 250 mrad/min
- Spot films: 50 mrad per spot film

EXAM

1 Obtain Informed Consent

Obtain informed consent from the patient or surrogate:

1. Risks: bleeding, infection, pain, headaches, seizures
2. Benefits
3. Alternatives

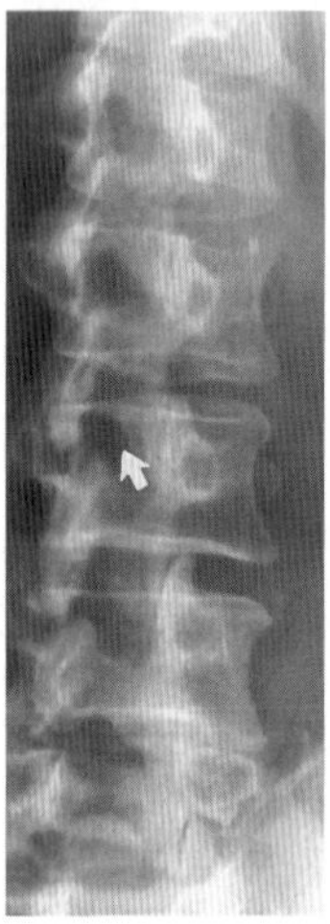

2 Localize Access Site

TABLETOP
Horizontal

75 kVp

PATIENT
LAO/RAO

Inspect the scout film for variant spinal anatomy and select the site of optimal access. Unless there is a contraindication, the L2-L3 interspace is often utilized because of an increased incidence of degenerative pathology at the lower lumbar levels. However, lumbar puncture at any lower lumbar level can be performed. Lumbar puncture should be avoided cephalad to L2 to prevent inadvertent injury to the cord.

Place the patient prone on the fluoroscopy table. Under fluoroscopic guidance, use a metal hemostat to localize the anticipated level of access. Slightly oblique the patient to allow visualization of a vertical course under the lamina into the thecal sac. Collimate as needed to focus on the spine.

Make a mark on the skin using a needle cap or a surgical marking pen at the site of anticipated puncture.

Alternatively, patients with laminectomies can be positioned prone and the thecal sac accessed with a midline puncture technique.

℞

3 Administer Local Anesthetic

TABLETOP
Horizontal

PATIENT
LAO/RAO

Using sterile technique, cleanse the overlying skin with povidone-iodine solution. Then wipe the anticipated puncture site with an alcohol swab.

Anesthetize with 1% lidocaine along the anticipated needle course.

4 Prepare Contrast

TABLETOP
Horizontal

PATIENT
LAO/RAO

Calculate the needed quantity of nonionic contrast material using the manufacturer's recommended dosing instructions. A 3.06 g limit of iodinated contrast is followed for adults.

Fill the 20 cc syringe with the needed volume of contrast; then attach it to the plastic extension tubing. Flush the tubing with contrast to expel all of the air from the system.

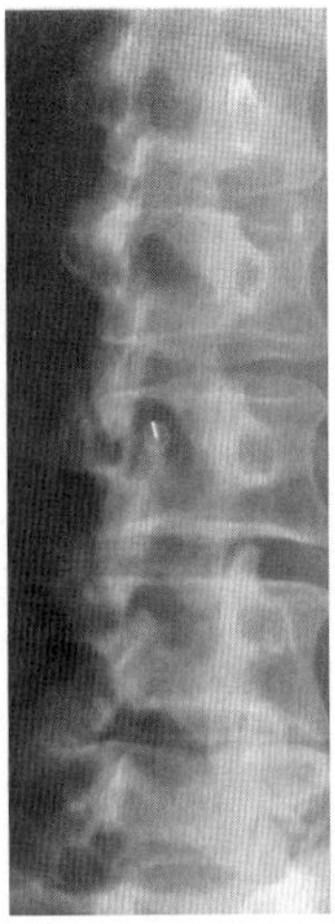

5 *Insert Spinal Needle*

Shallowly insert the spinal needle (with the stylet in place), keeping the notch on the needle hub directed perpendicular to the long axis of the spine so that the bevel of the needle will separate (not transect) the dural fibers.

The needle should be precisely positioned in both the horizontal and vertical axes so that it superimposes upon itself.

TABLETOP
Horizontal

PATIENT
LAO/RAO

6 *Access Thecal Sac*

Continue to advance the needle under intermittent fluoroscopic guidance into the soft tissues and verify that the needle is on course.

Elevate the patient's head to allow hydrostatic pressure to expand the thecal sac. Continue advancing the needle until the slight resistance of the ligamentum flavum is felt, followed by resistance of the dura, before entering the subarachnoid space. A second pop should be felt as the thecal sac is entered. The stylet should be periodically removed to check for the flow of cerebrospinal fluid. If there is no return of cerebrospinal fluid at the expected depth, a cross-table lateral film can be obtained to confirm correct needle placement.

TABLETOP
Head Up
15°

PATIENT
LAO/RAO

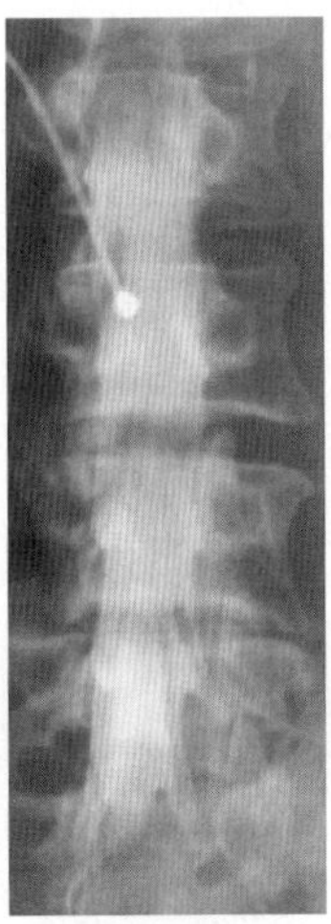

14 × 14
1 on 1
or
spot film

7 *Instill Contrast*

Cautiously connect the contrast-primed extension tubing to the spinal needle hub, making sure not to reposition the needle tip inadvertently.

With the patient in the prone position, slowly instill the contrast under intermittent fluoroscopic observation to determine the quantity needed to opacify the thecal sac. Keeping the tabletop in the 15° head upright position ensures accumulation of the contrast dependently.

It is important to establish that the contrast is being injected in a subarachnoid location. A visualized focal collection of contrast indicates aberrant epidural or subdural needle positioning.

Document the needle placement.

TABLETOP
Head Up
15°

PATIENT
PA

8 *Withdraw Spinal Needle*

Replace the stylet and carefully withdraw the spinal needle and stylet. Then clean the skin and cover the puncture site with antibiotic ointment and a small bandage.

TABLETOP
Horizontal

PATIENT
PA

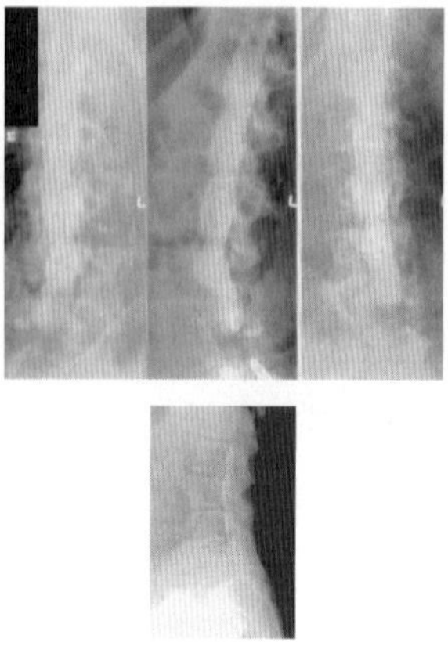

14 × 14
1–3 on 1

9 *Obtain Conventional Myelogram Films*

Obtain the following images of the lumbar spine and opacified thecal sac:

1. AP
2. LAO
3. RAO
4. Lateral

Standing flexion/extension lateral views may be beneficial to accentuate disk protrusions.

TABLETOP
Horizontal
± Vertical

PATIENT
AP
LAO
RAO
Lat

10 *Write Postprocedure Orders*

The patient should be directed to restrict activity for 24 hours, to drink plenty of fluids, and to avoid bending or heavy lifting. Restricted medications can be resumed after 24 hours. The head should be kept elevated to minimize intracranial flow of contrast.

11 *Obtain CT Myelogram*

Use the information obtained on the conventional myelogram to plan the postmyelographic CT protocol. ■

Cervical Myelogram

Cervical myelography is routinely performed with a combination of conventional imaging and CT after intrathecal administration of iodinated contrast.

The lateral C1-C2 puncture technique is an inherently dangerous procedure that should be performed only by radiologists specifically trained in this technique.

INDICATIONS

- Contraindication to MRI (e.g., pacemaker, aneurysm clip, claustrophobia, metal implants)
- Confirmation of equivocal MRI findings

CONTRAINDICATIONS

- Increased intracranial pressure
- Soft tissue infection at puncture site
- Coagulopathy (relative contraindication)
- Contrast allergy
- Anomalous vasculature (e.g., extracranial extension of posterior inferior cerebellar artery)

PATIENT PREPARATION

- NPO after midnight or 6 hours prior to exam
- Historically, medications that lower seizure threshold (e.g., phenothiazines, antipsychotics, tricyclic antidepressants, CNS stimulants, monoamine oxidase inhibitors, lithium, reserpine, isoniazid) have been discontinued 24–48 hours prior to nonemergent exams.

SUPPLIES

- Written consent form
- Metal hemostat
- Surgical marking pen
- Sterile gloves
- Nonionic contrast approved for myelography (e.g., Omnipaque 180/240/300, Isovue-M 200/300)
- 20 cc syringe (for contrast)
- 18 gauge needle (for drawing contrast)
- Povidone-iodine solution (e.g., Betadine)
- 3 prep swabs
- Alcohol swab
- Sterile 4 × 4 gauze
- Sterile fenestrated drape
- 5 cc 1% lidocaine without epinephrine
- 5 cc syringe (for lidocaine)
- 1½ inch 25 gauge needle (for lidocaine)
- 18 gauge needle (for drawing lidocaine)
- 3½ inch 22 gauge spinal needle with stylet
- Long plastic extension tubing
- Antibiotic ointment
- Small bandage

SCOUT FILM

- Complete cervical spine series
- ±PA lumbar spine (if the lumbar puncture technique will be used)

SAMPLE DICTATION

Informed and written consent was obtained from the patient. The risks (including bleeding, infection, and seizures), benefits, and alternatives to the exam were discussed. The patient was placed in the prone oblique position on the fluoroscopy table, and was prepared and draped in a sterile fashion. Local anesthesia was achieved using 1% lidocaine solution. The L2-L3 interspace was localized, and a 3½ inch 22 gauge spinal needle and stylet were advanced into the thecal sac under intermittent fluoroscopic guidance. Approximately 10 cc Isovue-M 300 was instilled into the thecal sac. The stylet was replaced, and the spinal needle was removed. Conventional cervical myelogram films were then obtained. There is no evidence of cervical nerve root compression or extradural impression upon the thecal sac. There were no immediate postprocedure complications. ■

RADIATION

- Fluoro: 50 mrad/min
- Spot films: 10 mrad per spot film

EXAM

1 *Obtain Consent*

Obtain informed consent from the patient or surrogate:

1. Risks: bleeding, infection, pain, headaches, seizures, stroke
2. Benefits
3. Alternatives

2 *Determine Lumbar or Cervical Approach*

Cervical myelography can be performed using either a lumbar or cervical approach.

The lumbar appoach is more common, as it is easier to gain access to the thecal sac, has a lower complication rate, and is generally preferred by patients. The disadvantages are that it can be difficult to control the movement of the contrast bolus to the cervical region, the contrast can be easily diluted, and some patients may have difficulty adequately hyperextending the neck, which is necessary when using the lumbar approach.

The cervical approach is technically more difficult to perform, especially without lateral fluoroscopy, and may result in cord puncture or vertebral artery laceration.

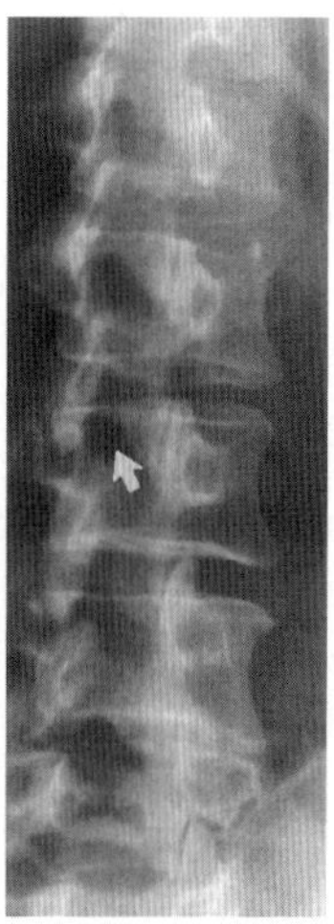

3a *Localize Access Site (Lumbar Approach)*

Inspect the scout film for variant spinal anatomy and select the site of optimal access. Unless there is a contraindication, the L2-L3 interspace is often utilized because of an increased incidence of degenerative pathology at the lower lumbar levels. However, lumbar puncture at any lower lumbar level can be performed. Lumbar puncture should be avoided cephalad to L2 to prevent inadvertent injury to the cord.

Place the patient prone on the fluoroscopy table. Under fluoroscopic guidance, use a metal hemostat to localize the anticipated level of access. Slightly oblique the patient to allow visualization of a vertical course under the lamina into the thecal sac. Collimate as needed to focus on the spine.

Make a mark on the skin using a needle cap or a surgical marking pen at the site of anticipated puncture.

Alternatively, patients with laminectomies can be positioned prone and the thecal sac accessed with a midline puncture technique.

TABLETOP

Horizontal

75 kVp

PATIENT

LAO/RAO

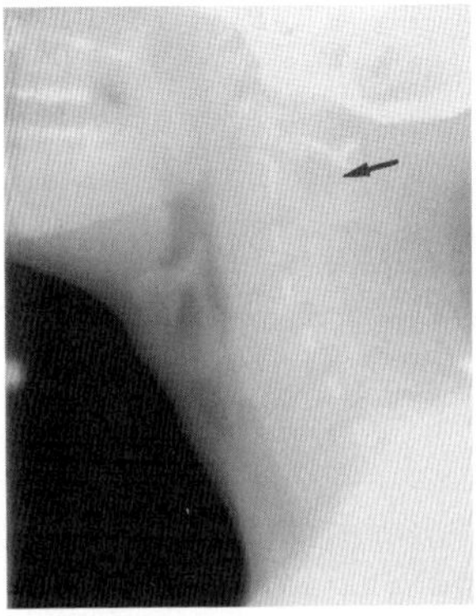

3b *Localize Access Site (Cervical Approach)*

The patient is placed in the prone position with the neck extended and is cautioned not to talk or move during the procedure.

Under lateral fluoroscopic visualization, verify the true lateral positioning by checking for superimposition of the mandibular condyles. Under fluoroscopic guidance, use a metal hemostat to localize the site of access just anterior to the spinolaminal line at the C1-C2 level.

If lateral fluoroscopy is not available, the C1-C2 puncture can be performed with the patient in the true lateral position.

Make a mark on the skin using a needle cap or a surgical marking pen at the site of anticipated puncture.

TABLETOP
Horizontal

75 kVp

PATIENT
PA

℞

4 *Administer Local Anesthetic*

Using sterile technique, cleanse the overlying skin with povidone-iodine solution. Then wipe the anticipated puncture site with an alcohol swab.

Anesthetize with 1% lidocaine along the anticipated needle course.

TABLETOP
Horizontal

PATIENT
PA/LAO/RAO

5 *Prepare Contrast*

Calculate the needed quantity of nonionic contrast material using the manufacturer's recommended dosing instructions. A 3.06 g limit of iodinated contrast is followed for adults.

Nonionic contrast containing 180–240 mg I/mL is generally used for adult cervical myelography with a lateral C1-C2 approach, while contrast containing 200–300 mg I/mL is used with a lumbar approach.

Fill the 20 cc syringe with the needed volume of contrast; then attach it to the plastic extension tubing. Flush the tubing with contrast to expel all of the air from the system.

TABLETOP
Horizontal

PATIENT
PA/LAO/RAO

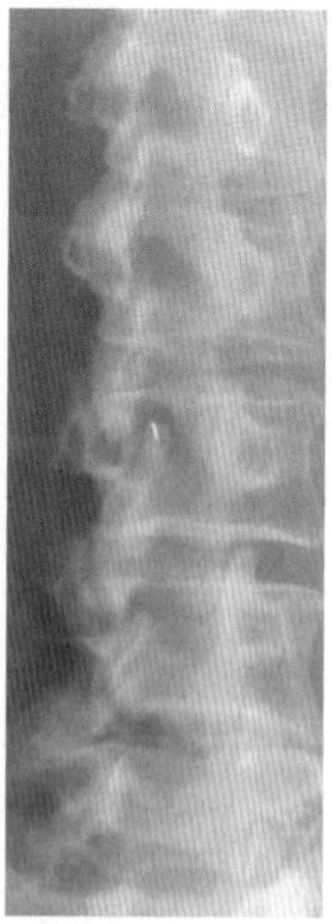

6a *Perform Lumbar Puncture*

Shallowly insert the spinal needle (with the stylet in place), keeping the notch on the needle hub directed perpendicular to the long axis of the spine so that the bevel of the needle will separate (not transect) the dural fibers.

The needle should be precisely positioned in both the horizontal and vertical axes so that it superimposes upon itself.

Continue to advance the needle under intermittent fluoroscopic guidance into the soft tissues and verify that the needle is on course.

Elevate the patient's head to allow hydrostatic pressure to expand the thecal sac. Continue advancing the needle until the slight resistance of the ligamentum flavum is felt, followed by resistance of the dura, before entering the subarachnoid space. A second pop should be felt as the thecal sac is entered. The stylet should be periodically removed to check for the flow of cerebrospinal fluid. If there is no return of cerebrospinal fluid at the expected depth, a cross-table lateral film can be obtained to confirm correct needle placement.

TABLETOP

Horizontal/

Head Up 20°

75 kVp

PATIENT

LAO/RAO

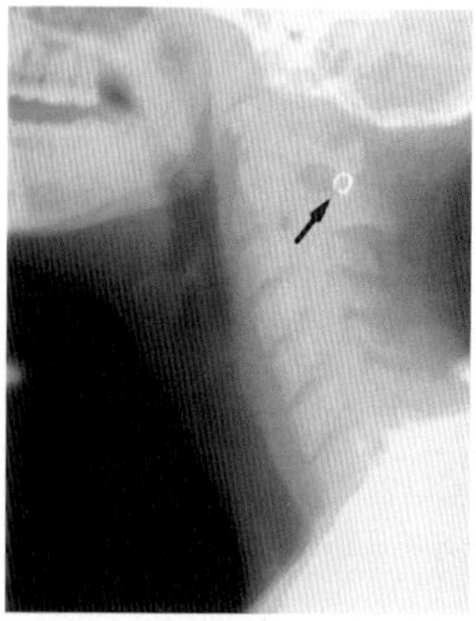

6b *Perform Lateral C1-C2 Puncture*

From a lateral puncture site, insert a 22 gauge spinal needle just anterior to the spinolaminal line at the C1-C2 level. Under PA fluoroscopic visualization, the needle tip should project just medial to the lateral margin of the dens.

Slowly advance the needle into the thecal sac, removing the stylet every 1–2 mm to check for cerebrospinal fluid flow once an appropriate depth is approached. At this level, blood return can be encountered when the epidural venous plexus is traversed. The resistance of the dura should be felt before entering the subarachnoid space. To avoid puncturing the cord, it is usually unnecessary to proceed anteriorly farther than the posterior third of the spinal canal.

TABLETOP

Horizontal

75 kVp

PATIENT

PA

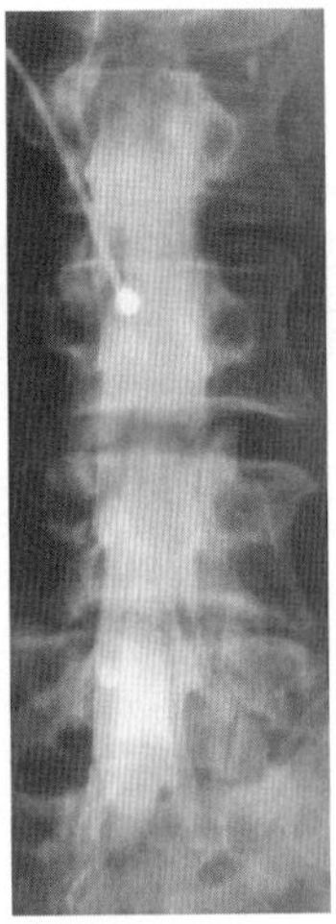

14 × 14
1 on 1
or
spot film

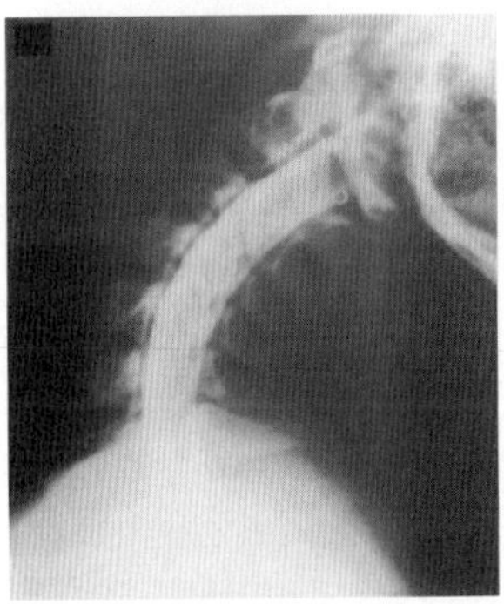

10 × 12
1 on 1
or
spot film

7 *Instill Contrast*

Cautiously connect the contrast-primed extension tubing to the spinal needle hub, making sure not to reposition the needle tip inadvertently.

Instill the contrast under intermittent fluoroscopic observation to determine the quantity needed to opacify the thecal sac. It is important to establish that the contrast is being injected in a subarachnoid location. A visualized focal collection of contrast indicates epidural, subdural, spinal cord, or other aberrant needle positioning. Gradually elevate the head of the table to prevent intracranial flow of contrast.

If a lumbar puncture was utilized, the maximum contrast load should be administered and delivered to the cervical spine as a bolus by placing the patient in the Trendelenburg position. It is sometimes necessary to place the patient in a very steep head-down or lateral position to guide the contrast beyond the thoracic kyphosis. The patient's neck should be hyperextended to prevent intracranial passage of contrast. Once contrast reaches the cervical region, the patient should be returned to the horizontal prone position. The contrast will subsequently pool in the cervical thecal sac because of the natural cervical lordosis.

Document the needle placement.

TABLETOP
Various

PATIENT
PA

8 *Withdraw Spinal Needle*

Replace the stylet and carefully withdraw the spinal needle and stylet. Then clean the skin and cover the puncture site with antibiotic ointment and a small bandage.

TABLETOP
Horizontal

PATIENT
PA

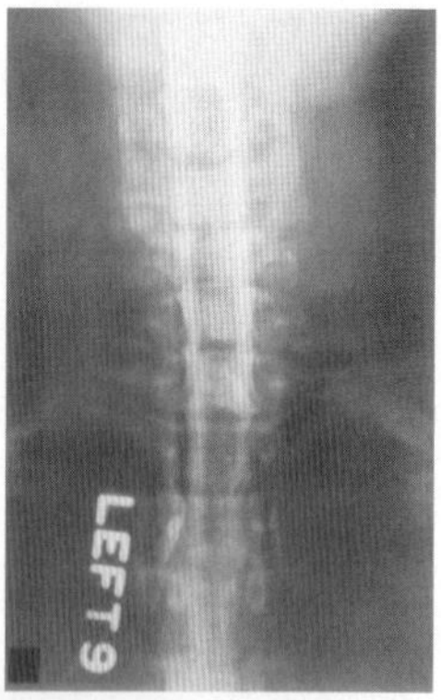

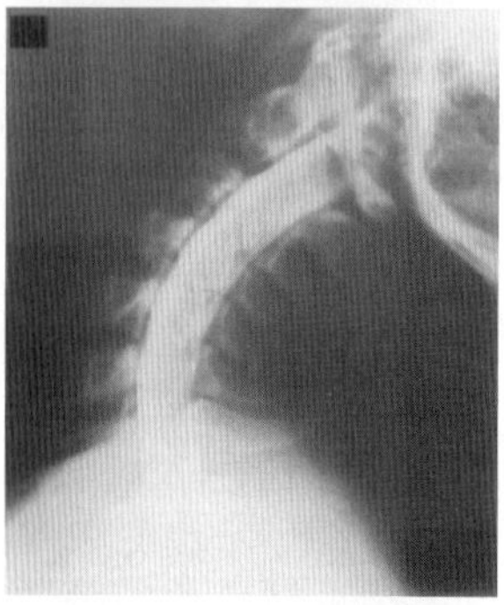

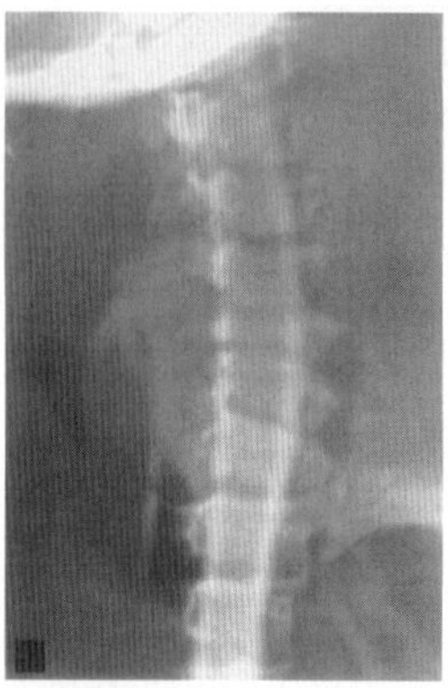

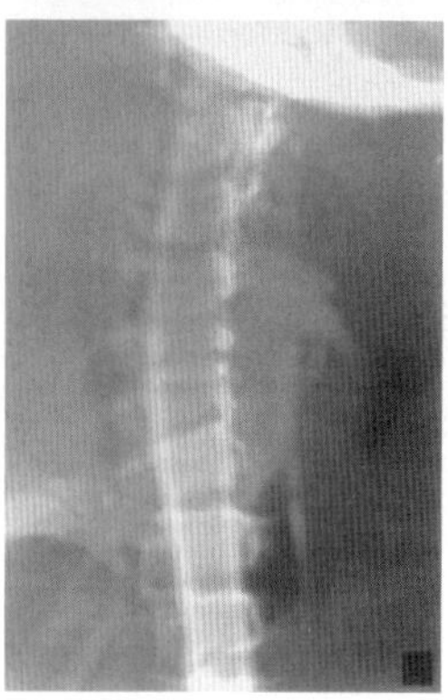

9 *Obtain Conventional Myelograms*

Obtain the following overhead images (within 2–3 minutes for optimum visualization) of the conventional myelogram with the tube angled 20–30° cephalad to delineate the nerve roots:

1. AP
2. Lateral
3. LAO
4. RAO
5. Swimmer's

(Images from Orrison WW: Introduction to Neuroimaging. *Boston: Little, Brown and Company, 1989, p. 310; reprinted by permission of Lippincott Williams & Wilkins.)*

TABLETOP

Horizontal

PATIENT

AP

Lat

LAO

RAO

Swimmer's

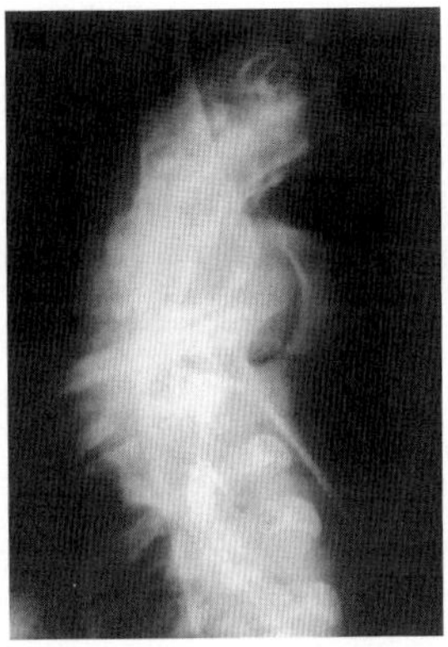

10 × 12
1 on 1

9 *Obtain Conventional Myelograms* *(continued)*

10 *Write Postprocedure Orders*

The patient should be directed to restrict activity for 24 hours and to avoid bending or heavy lifting. Restricted medications can be resumed after 24 hours. The head should be kept elevated to minimize intracranial flow of contrast. Hydration should be encouraged.

11 *Obtain CT Myelogram*

Use the information obtained on the conventional myelogram to guide the CT myelogram. ■

Thoracic Myelogram

Thoracic myelography is routinely performed with a combination of conventional imaging and CT after intrathecal administration of iodinated contrast.

INDICATIONS

- Contraindication to MRI (e.g., pacemaker, claustrophobia, metal implants)
- Confirmation of equivocal MRI findings

CONTRAINDICATIONS

- Increased intracranial pressure
- Soft tissue infection at puncture site
- Coagulopathy (relative contraindication)
- Contrast allergy

PATIENT PREPARATION

- NPO after midnight or 6 hours prior to exam
- Historically, medications that lower seizure threshold (e.g., phenothiazines, antipsychotics, tricyclic antidepressants, CNS stimulants, monoamine oxidase inhibitors, lithium, reserpine, isoniazid) have been discontinued 24–48 hours prior to nonemergent exams.

SUPPLIES

- Written consent form
- Metal hemostat
- Surgical marking pen
- Sterile gloves
- Nonionic contrast approved for myelography (e.g., Omnipaque 240/300, Isovue-M 200/300)
- 20 cc syringe (for contrast)
- 18 gauge needle (for drawing contrast)
- Povidone-iodine solution (e.g., Betadine)
- 3 prep swabs
- Alcohol swab
- Sterile 4 × 4 gauze
- Sterile fenestrated drape
- 5 cc 1% lidocaine without epinephrine
- 5 cc syringe (for lidocaine)
- 1½ inch 25 gauge needle (for lidocaine)
- 18 gauge needle (for drawing lidocaine)
- 3½ inch 22 gauge spinal needle with stylet
- Long plastic extension tubing
- Antibiotic ointment
- Small bandage

SCOUT FILM

- Complete thoracic spine series
- PA lumbar spine

SAMPLE DICTATION

Informed and written consent was obtained from the patient. The risks (including bleeding, infection, and seizures), benefits, and alternatives to the exam were discussed. The patient was placed in the prone oblique position on the fluoroscopy table, and was prepared and draped in a sterile fashion. Local anesthesia was achieved using 1% lidocaine solution. The L2-L3 interspace was localized, and a 3½ inch 22 gauge spinal needle and stylet were advanced into the thecal sac under intermittent fluoroscopic guidance. Approximately 10 cc Isovue-M 200 was instilled into the thecal sac. The stylet was replaced, and the spinal needle was removed. Conventional thoracic myelogram films were then obtained. There is no evidence of thoracic nerve root compression or extradural impression upon the thecal sac. There were no immediate postprocedure complications. ■

RADIATION

- Fluoro: 250 mrad/min
- Spot films: 50 mrad per spot film

EXAM

1 *Obtain Informed Consent*

Obtain informed consent from the patient or surrogate:

1. Risks: bleeding, infection, pain, headaches, seizures
2. Benefits
3. Alternatives

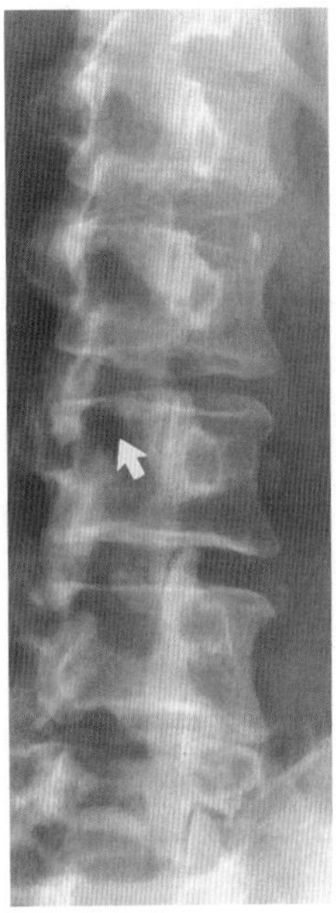

2 *Localize Access Site*

Inspect the scout film for variant spinal anatomy and select the site of optimal access. Unless there is a contraindication, the L2-L3 interspace is often utilized because of an increased incidence of degenerative pathology at the lower lumbar levels. However, lumbar puncture at any lower lumbar level can be performed. Lumbar puncture should be avoided cephalad to L2 to prevent inadvertent injury to the cord.

Place the patient prone on the fluoroscopy table. Under fluoroscopic guidance, use a metal hemostat to localize the anticipated level of access. Slightly oblique the patient to allow visualization of a vertical course under the lamina into the thecal sac. Collimate as needed to focus on the spine.

Make a mark on the skin using a needle cap or a surgical marking pen at the site of anticipated puncture.

Alternatively, patients with laminectomies can be positioned prone and the thecal sac accessed with a midline puncture technique.

TABLETOP
Horizontal

75 kVp

PATIENT
LAO/RAO

℞

3 *Administer Local Anesthetic*

Using sterile technique, cleanse the overlying skin with povidone-iodine solution. Then wipe the anticipated puncture site with an alcohol swab.

Anesthetize with 1% lidocaine along the anticipated needle course.

TABLETOP
Horizontal

PATIENT
LAO/RAO

4 *Prepare Contrast*

Calculate the needed quantity of nonionic contrast material using the manufacturer's recommended dosing instructions. A 3.06 g limit of iodinated contrast is followed for adults.

Fill the 20 cc syringe with the needed volume of contrast; then attach it to the plastic extension tubing. Flush the tubing with contrast to expel all of the air from the system.

TABLETOP
Horizontal

PATIENT
LAO/RAO

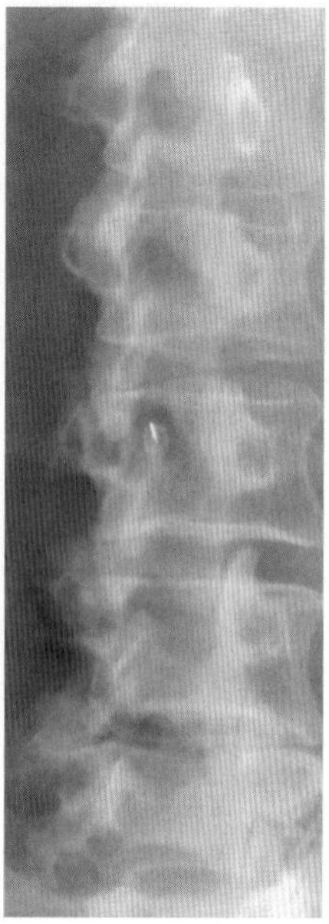

5 *Insert Spinal Needle*

Shallowly insert the spinal needle (with the stylet in place), keeping the notch on the needle hub directed perpendicular to the long axis of the spine so that the bevel of the needle will separate (not transect) the dural fibers.

The needle should be precisely positioned in both the horizontal and vertical axes so that it superimposes upon itself.

TABLETOP
Horizontal

PATIENT
LAO/RAO

6 *Access Thecal Sac*

Continue to advance the needle under intermittent fluoroscopic guidance into the soft tissues and verify that the needle is on course.

Elevate the patient's head to allow hydrostatic pressure to expand the thecal sac. Continue advancing the needle until the slight resistance of the ligamentum flavum is felt, followed by resistance of the dura, before entering the subarachnoid space. A second pop should be felt as the thecal sac is entered. The stylet should be periodically removed to check for the flow of cerebrospinal fluid. If there is no return of cerebrospinal fluid at the expected depth, a cross-table lateral film can be obtained to confirm correct needle placement.

TABLETOP
Head Up
15°

PATIENT
LAO/RAO

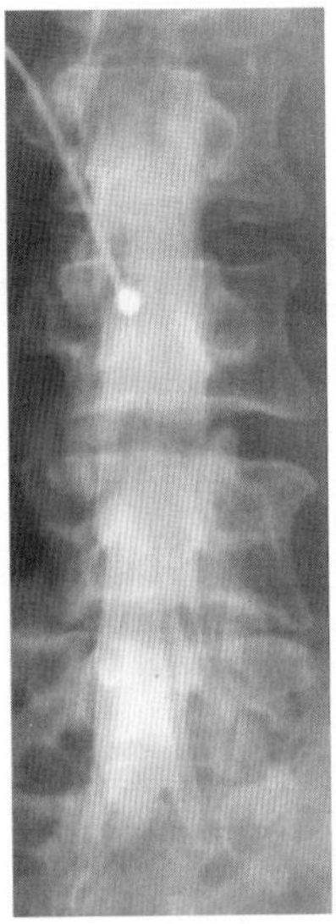

14 × 14
1 on 1
or
spot film

7 *Instill Contrast*

Cautiously connect the contrast-primed extension tubing to the spinal needle hub, making sure not to reposition the needle tip inadvertently.

With the patient in the prone position, slowly instill the contrast under intermittent fluoroscopic observation to determine the quantity needed to opacify the thecal sac. Keeping the tabletop in the 15° head-upright position ensures accumulation of the contrast dependently.

It is important to establish that the contrast is being injected in a subarachnoid location. A visualized focal collection of contrast indicates aberrant epidural or subdural needle positioning.

Document the needle placement.

TABLETOP
Head Up
15°

PATIENT
PA

8 *Withdraw Spinal Needle*

Replace the stylet and carefully withdraw the spinal needle and stylet. Then clean the skin and cover the puncture site with antibiotic ointment and a small bandage.

TABLETOP
Horizontal

PATIENT
PA

9 *Pool Contrast in Thoracic Region*

Gently roll the patient into the lateral or supine position, with the head remaining elevated. Under fluoroscopic visualization, decline the table to −15° and follow the contrast bolus into the thoracic region, smoothly manipulating the table position as necessary to pool the contrast in the desired location.

TABLETOP
Head Down
−15°

PATIENT
PA/Lat

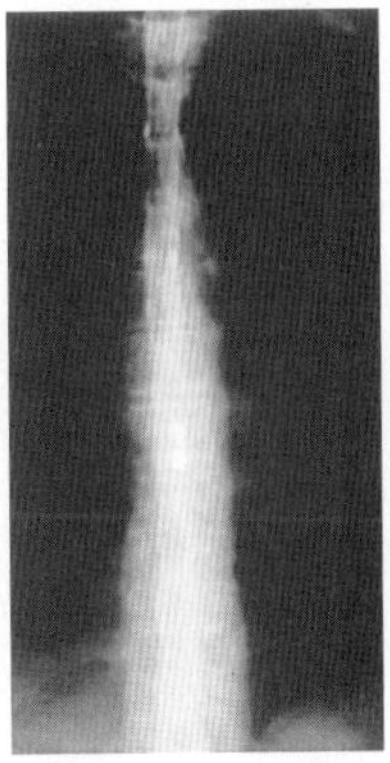

10 *Obtain Conventional Myelograms*

Obtain the following images of the thoracic spine and opacified thecal sac:

1. AP
2. Lateral
3. Swimmer's

Standing flexion/extension lateral views may be beneficial to accentuate disk protrusions.

TABLETOP
Head Down
−15°

PATIENT
AP
Lat
Swimmer's

↓

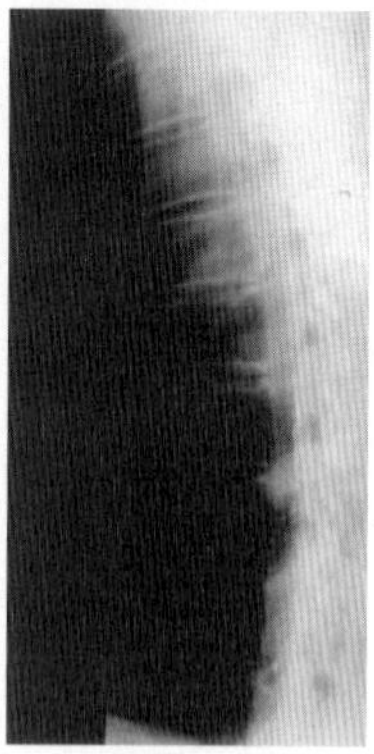

14 × 14
1–3 on 1

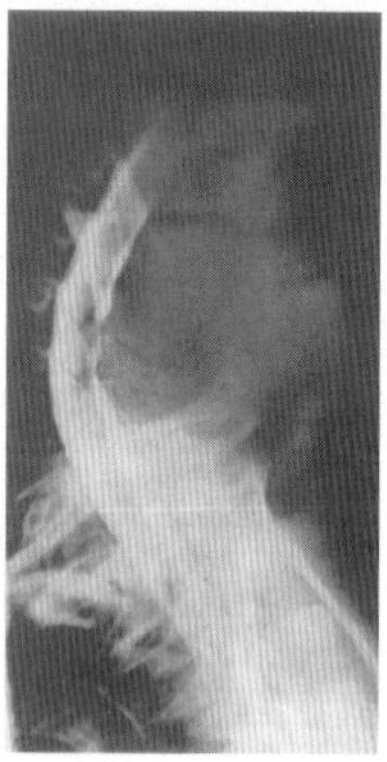

10 × 12
1 on 1

10 *Obtain Conventional Myelograms* *(continued)*

11 *Write Postprocedure Orders*

The patient should be directed to restrict activity for 24 hours and to avoid bending or heavy lifting. Restricted medications can be resumed after 24 hours. The head should be kept elevated to minimize intracranial flow of contrast. Hydration should be encouraged.

12 *Obtain CT Myelogram*

Use the information obtained on the conventional myelogram to guide the CT myelogram. ■

PART VIII
Pediatric Examinations

Jeffrey D. Houston, M.D.
Philip W. Wiest, M.D.

Pediatric Videofluoroscopic Swallowing Exam

INDICATIONS

- Dysphagia (difficulty swallowing)
- Suspected aspiration

CONTRAINDICATIONS

- If pharyngeal perforation is suspected, water-soluble contrast is used by convention.
- If aspiration or a fistula to the airway is suspected, ionic water-soluble contrast is avoided.

PATIENT PREPARATION

- NPO 2–4 hours (depending on age) prior to exam to stimulate appetite

SUPPLIES

- 2–4 oz regular barium (60% w/v)
- Bottle
- Variety of nipples
- Scalpel (for enlarging nipple opening)
- Suction should be available if the patient is unable to clear the airway of aspirated contents.
- ±60 cc catheter tip syringe

SCOUT FILM

- AP babygram

SAMPLE DICTATION

Videofluoroscopic swallowing evaluation was performed using regular barium. Oral transit was normal. There was no evidence of nasopharyngeal reflux, laryngeal penetration, or frank tracheal aspiration. No cricopharyngeal abnormalities were noted. The pharynx and cervical spine have a normal appearance. ■

RADIATION

- Pulsed fluoro: 325 mrad/min

EXAM

1 *Prepare Video Recorder*

Record the entire exam on videotape.

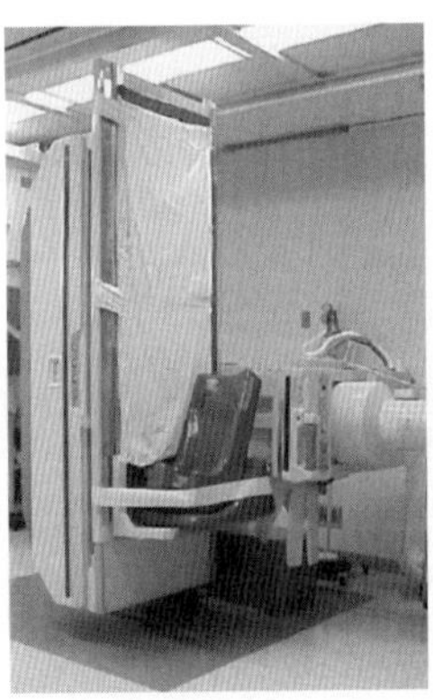

2 *Position Patient*

The patient is usually secured in a pediatric restraining chair. The restraining chair is placed in the right lateral position on the fluoroscope footboard and secured.

Select a nipple that closely resembles the type that the patient is accustomed to using. Enlarge the nipple opening to facilitate flow of contrast.

TABLETOP

Vertical

PATIENT

Rt Lat

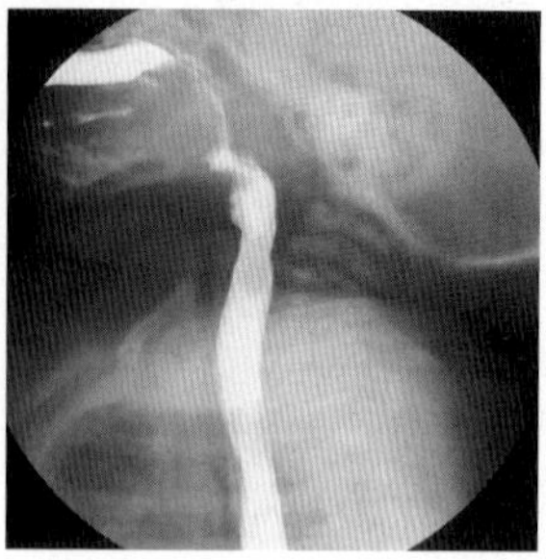

3 *Record Lateral Swallow*

Instruct an assistant, usually a family member, to hold the bottle for the patient to ensure optimal positioning. Position the fluoroscope to allow visualization of the mouth, pharynx, and cervical esophagus. This sequence is the most diagnostic and should be imaged first in case the patient is unable to continue with the examination. Multiple swallows are routinely imaged to permit assessment for fatigue.

If the patient will not use the nipple, barium can be injected into the mouth with a syringe.

Observation of swallowing in the AP projection is not routinely performed in the pediatric population, as it generally does not provide sufficient additional information to justify the increased radiation exposure. The AP projection should be obtained only if needed.

TABLETOP

Vertical

Pulsed fluoro

7.5 fr/sec

80 kVp

PATIENT

Rt Lat

±AP

4 *Perform Single Contrast UGI Series*

(see p. 175)

The swallowing examination is often followed by a single contrast UGI series with assessment for gastroesophageal reflux. ■

Pediatric Speech Pathology Swallowing Exam

INDICATIONS

- Dysphagia (difficulty swallowing)
- Suspected aspiration
- Laryngomalacia

CONTRAINDICATIONS

- Sufficient sedation to impede normal swallowing

PATIENT PREPARATION

- NPO 2–4 hours (depending on age) prior to exam to stimulate appetite

SUPPLIES

- 2–4 oz regular barium (60% w/v)
- 2–4 oz dense barium (200–250% w/v)
- Bottle
- Variety of nipples
- Scalpel (for enlarging nipple opening)
- ±60 cc catheter tip syringe
- Liquid thickener
- Assortment of foods mixed with barium paste (60–70% w/v)
- Plastic cutlery
- Suction should be available if the patient is unable to clear the airway of aspirated contents.

SCOUT FILM

- AP babygram

SAMPLE DICTATION

Videofluoroscopic swallowing examination was performed in conjunction with the speech pathology department. Various liquid and solid food substances were used to assess the patient's swallowing mechanism. The patient swallowed liquid barium of various consistencies, as well as semisolid and solid food substances without difficulty. No tracheal aspiration was noted. ■

RADIATION

- Pulsed fluoro: 325 mrad/min

EXAM

1 *Prepare Video Recorder*

Record the entire exam on videotape.

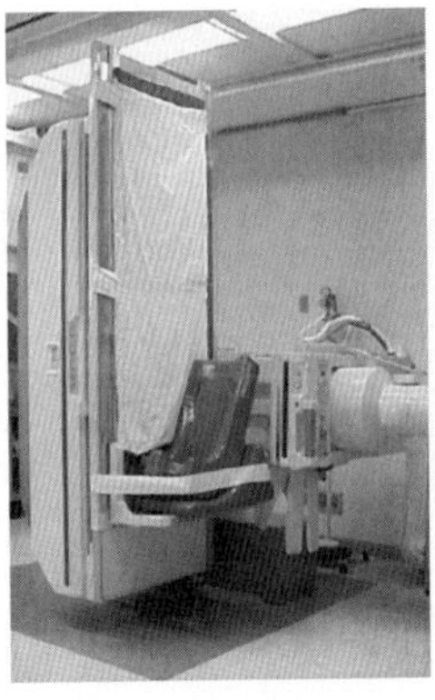

2 *Position Patient*

The patient is usually secured in a pediatric restraining chair. The restraining chair is placed in the right lateral position on the fluoroscope footboard and secured.

Select a nipple that closely resembles the type that the patient is accustomed to using. Enlarge the nipple opening to facilitate the flow of contrast.

TABLETOP

Vertical

PATIENT

Rt Lat

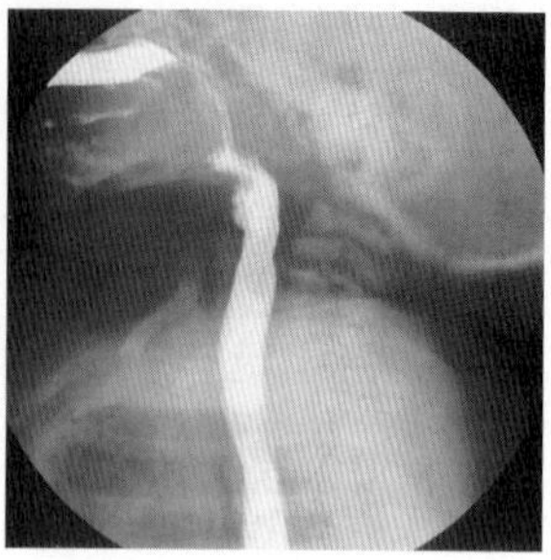

3 Record Lateral Swallow

Center the fluoroscope over the mouth and pharynx. The speech pathologist will administer small volumes of the designated substance to the patient.

Observe for the following findings:

1. Quality of oral transfer
2. Pooling in valleculae and pyriform recesses
3. Nasopharyngeal reflux
4. Laryngeal penetration
5. Frank tracheal aspiration (below true cords)
6. Cricopharyngeal hypertrophy
7. Posterior pharyngeal wall thickening (edema, hematoma, abscess)

If significant aspiration occurs, terminate the exam.

TABLETOP
Vertical

Pulsed fluoro
7.5 fr/sec
80 kVp

PATIENT
Rt Lat

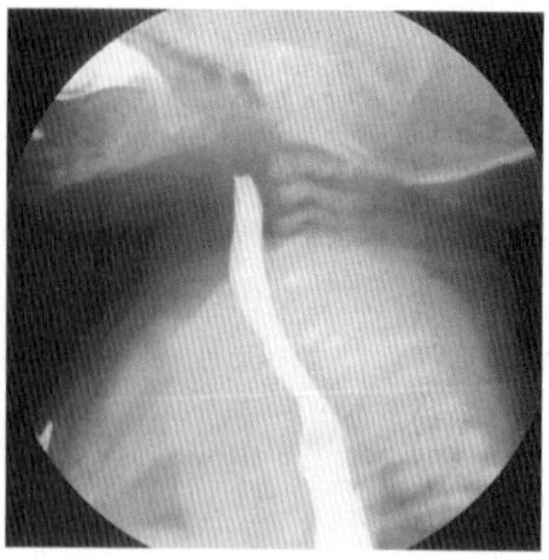

4 Record Repeat Swallows

The subsequent swallows follow the same sequence, except that different food substances mixed with barium are used. Common foods include:

1. Thinned barium
2. Thickened barium
3. Applesauce
4. Pudding
5. Cheese
6. Cookies
7. Sliced meat
8. Carbonated beverages
9. Ice

If the speech pathologist desires, the pediatric restraining chair can be rotated into the AP position and additional swallows observed in this projection. ■

TABLETOP
Vertical

PATIENT
Rt Lat
±AP

Pediatric Single Contrast Upper Gastrointestinal Series

INDICATIONS

- Suspected gastroesophageal reflux
- Suspected malrotation and midgut volvulus
- Evaluation of masses, vascular rings/slings, strictures, or aberrant anatomy
- Suspected hypertrophic pyloric stenosis (ultrasound is often preferred)

CONTRAINDICATIONS

- Suspected perforation of viscus (use water-soluble contrast)
- If aspiration or a fistula to the airway is suspected, ionic water-soluble contrast is avoided.
- Suspected esophageal atresia with tracheoesophageal fistula (perform bronchoscopy)

PATIENT PREPARATION

- NPO 2–4 hours (depending on age) prior to exam to stimulate appetite

SUPPLIES

- 2–8 oz regular barium (60% w/v)
- Bottle
- Variety of nipples
- Scalpel (for enlarging nipple opening)
- ±Pediatric nasograstric/orogastric tube
- ±60 cc catheter tip syringe

SCOUT FILM

- Not obtained routinely

SAMPLE DICTATION

Normal esophageal motility is present. There is no evidence of esophageal masses, strictures, ulcerations, or other abnormalities. The stomach has a normal appearance. Normal gastric emptying was observed. The duodenojejunal junction is normally positioned. No gastroesophageal reflux was identified during 5 minutes of intermittent fluoroscopic observation. ■

RADIATION

- Pulsed fluoro: 325 mrad/min
- Spot films: 50 mrad per spot film
  Digital spot films are preferred over cassettes to reduce radiation exposure.

TABLE 1. *Maximum Number of Episodes of Gastroesophageal Reflux Allowed During 5 Minutes of Observation*

AGE	MAXIMUM EPISODES OF REFLUX
Birth–6 weeks	3
6 weeks–1 year	2
1 year–6 years	1
6–18 years	0–1

EXAM

1 *Position Patient*

A nipple should be selected that closely resembles the type that the patient is accustomed to using. The nipple opening should be enlarged to facilitate the flow of contrast.

Place the patient in the right lateral position between two sandbags. Instruct an assistant, usually a family member, to hold the bottle for the patient to ensure optimal positioning.

TABLETOP

Horizontal

PATIENT

Rt Lat

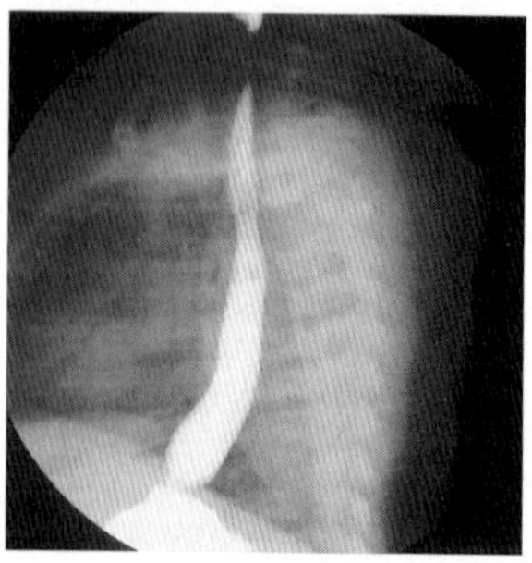

spot film

2 *Image Lateral Esophagus*

Position the fluoroscope to allow visualization of the mouth, pharynx, and cervical esophagus. Observe the swallowing mechanism. Then obtain images of the entire esophagus as it becomes distended with contrast.

If the patient will not use the nipple, barium can be injected into the mouth with a syringe. If the patient will not swallow, an orogastric or nasogastric tube may need to be placed in the proximal esophagus.

TABLETOP

Horizontal

Pulsed fluoro

7.5 fr/sec

80 kVp

PATIENT

Rt Lat

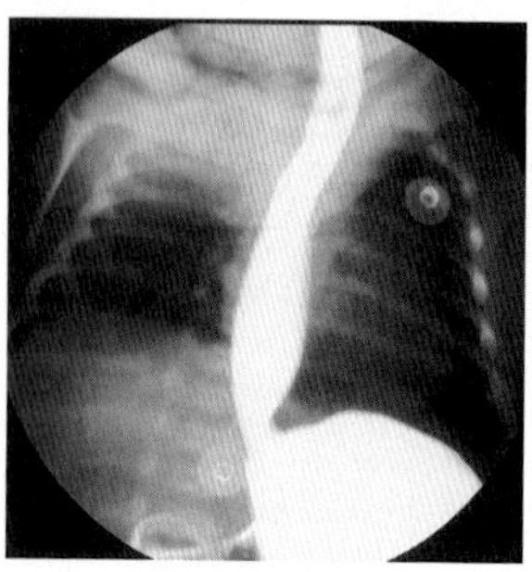

spot film

3 *Image AP Esophagus*

After a sufficient number of swallows have been observed in the lateral position, the patient is moved into the supine position. An assistant should again hold the bottle for the patient to ensure optimal positioning. The bottle should be held slightly to the side to avoid obscuring the esophagus.

Obtain images of the entire esophagus as it becomes distended with contrast.

TABLETOP

Horizontal

PATIENT

AP

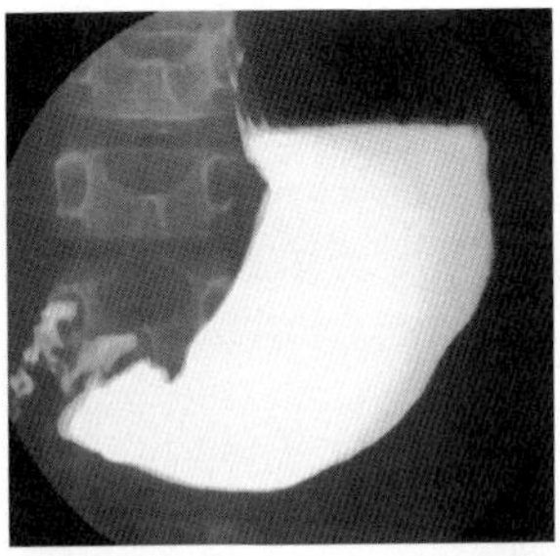

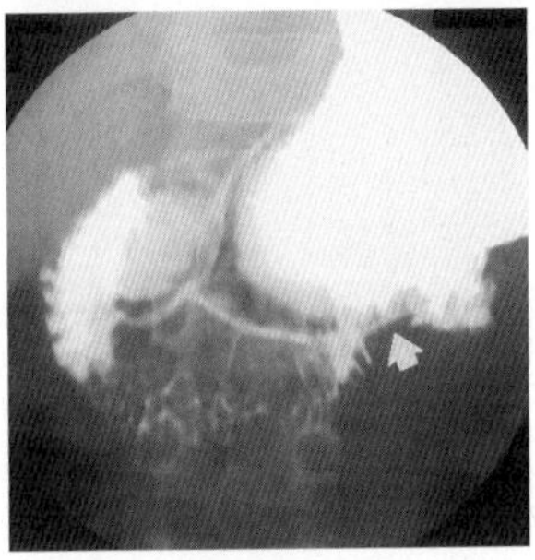

spot film

4 *Image AP Stomach and Duodenum*

Image the filled stomach and duodenum, documenting the position of the duodenojejunal junction. The duodenojejunal junction should normally project over the left L1 pedicle at the same level as the pylorus.

TABLETOP

Horizontal

PATIENT

AP

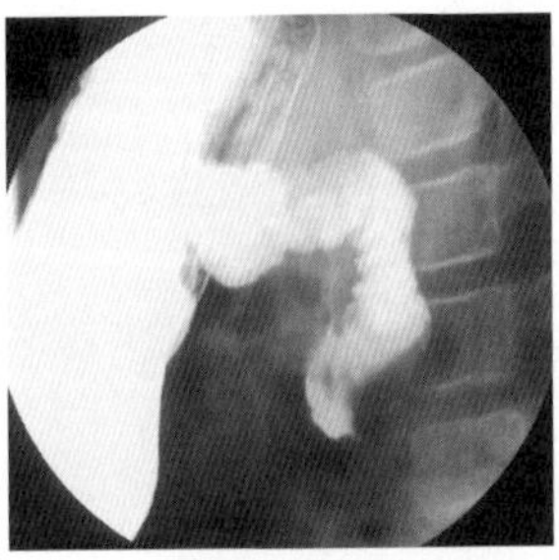

spot film

5 *Image Lateral Stomach and Duodenum*

Image the distended duodenum and document the position of the duodenojejunal junction.

TABLETOP

Horizontal

PATIENT

Rt Lat

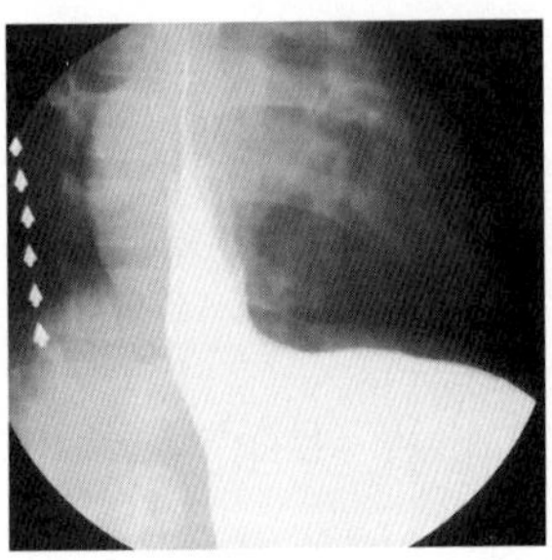

spot film

6 *Observe for Gastroesophageal Reflux*

Place an adhesive radiopaque marker on the image intensifier to indicate that subsequent images represent gastroesophageal reflux.

If a sufficient quantity of contrast has not been consumed, the patient can be fed milk, formula, juice, or water to increase the gastric volume. The patient should be burped if the stomach is significantly distended with air. ↓

TABLETOP

Horizontal

PATIENT

AP

6 *Observe for Gastroesophageal Reflux* *(continued)*

The esophagus should be fluoroscopically observed approximately every few seconds for 5 minutes to assess for gastroesophageal reflux. If reflux is observed, spot films should be obtained for documentation and assessment of severity. Reflux around an orogastric or nasogastric tube is not considered abnormal. Thus tube removal is often necessary to assess for pathologic reflux.

It is imperative that the patient not be upset during the examination, as crying increases intrathoracic pressure and negates gastroesophageal reflux. An assistant can occupy the child's attention or toys can be offered to older children to keep them calm.

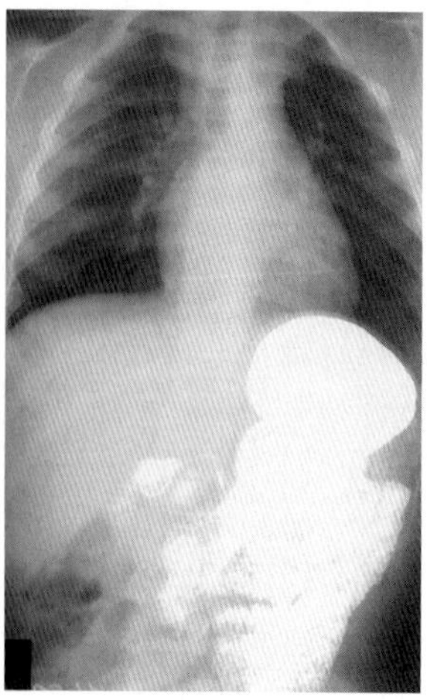

10 × 12
or
30 × 35 cm

7 *Obtain Overhead Film(s)*

Have the technologist obtain an overhead AP babygram or abdomen film, depending on age, and additional films as needed. ■

TABLETOP

Horizontal

80 kVp

PATIENT

AP

Pediatric Single Contrast Enema

INDICATIONS

- Neonatal distal bowel obstruction
- Distal colon study before colostomy takedown
- Hirschsprung disease (see specific instructions below)

CONTRAINDICATIONS

- Perforation
- Pneumatosis (relative)
- Hemodynamic instability

PATIENT PREPARATION

- A bowel prep is not generally necessary
- ±Intravenous access for fluid administration (contrast will dehydrate patient)

SUPPLIES

- 200 cc 20% diatrizoate sodium solution (e.g., Hypaque Sodium Oral Powder)
- Barium enema bag with tubing
- Thin and wide tape
- Variety of pediatric enema tips
- Lubrication jelly

SCOUT FILM

- AP babygram

SAMPLE DICTATION

The entire colon was filled with 20% Hypaque solution, and contrast was refluxed into the terminal ileum. The colon is normal in caliber throughout. No strictures, masses, or other abnormalities are seen. The cecum is normally positioned in the right lower quadrant. ■

RADIATION

- Pulsed fluoro: 325 mrad/min
- Spot films: 50 mrad per spot film
  Digital spot films are preferred over cassettes to reduce radiation exposure.

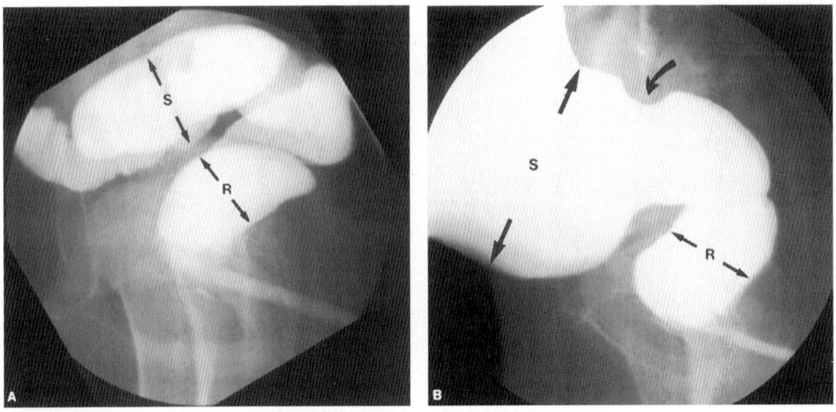

arrow—transition zone (in Hirschsprung disease)
S—sigmoid diameter
R—rectal diameter

FIGURE 1. *Normal (A) and abnormal (B) rectosigmoid indices. The rectosigmoid index (maximum dimension of rectum/maximum dimension of sigmoid) is normally 1.0 or greater.*

EXAM

1 *Insert Enema Tip in Rectum*

Connect the enema tip to the tubing and flush the tubing with contrast to express any remaining air. Select the smallest enema tip that will fit the patient. Gently insert the lubricated enema tip into the rectum. Using a combination of thin and wide tape, secure the tube to the skin and tape the buttocks together to form a seal around the enema tip. Immobilize the patient between two sandbags.

TABLETOP
Horizontal

Pulsed fluoro
7.5 fr/sec
80 kVp

PATIENT
PA

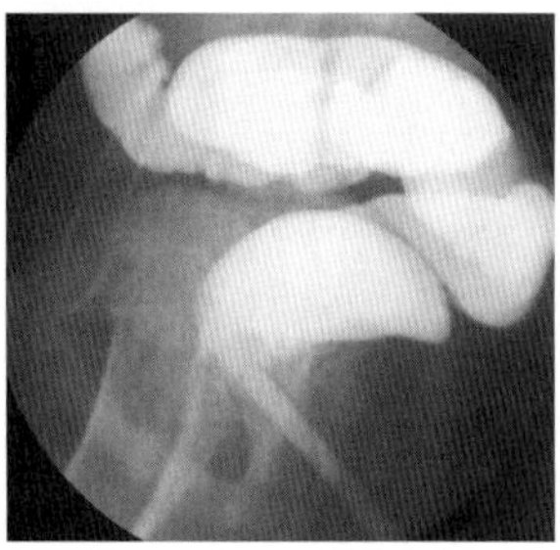

spot film

2 *Image Lateral Rectum*

Slowly fill the rectum with contrast while observing under fluoroscopy. Image the distended lateral rectum. Terminate filling with contrast if a perforation is encountered or if an abnormal rectosigmoid index is identified. The rectosigmoid index is calculated on the lateral view:

$$\text{Rectosigmoid Index} = \frac{\text{Maximum dimension of rectum}}{\text{Maximum dimension of sigmoid}}$$

Normally the rectum is wider than the sigmoid colon at their widest points and the ratio is 1.0 or greater.

TABLETOP
Horizontal

PATIENT
Lat

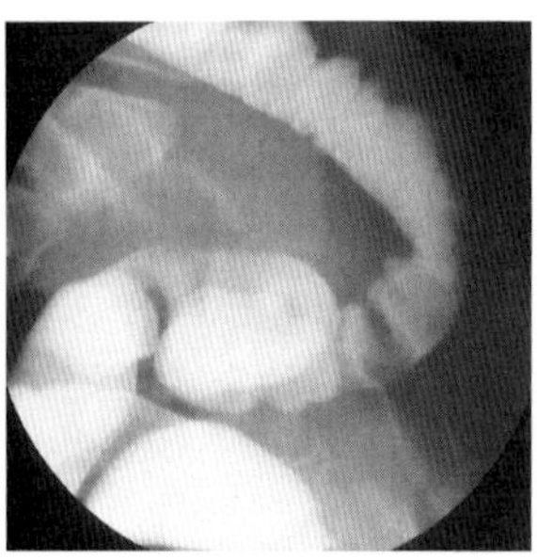

3 *Image Remainder of Colon*

With the patient in the supine position, continue filling the colon with contrast and acquire representative spot images as the colonic segments fill. Terminate filling once contrast is refluxed into the terminal ileum or a colostomy/mucus fistula site is reached.

TABLETOP
Horizontal

PATIENT
AP
±Obliques

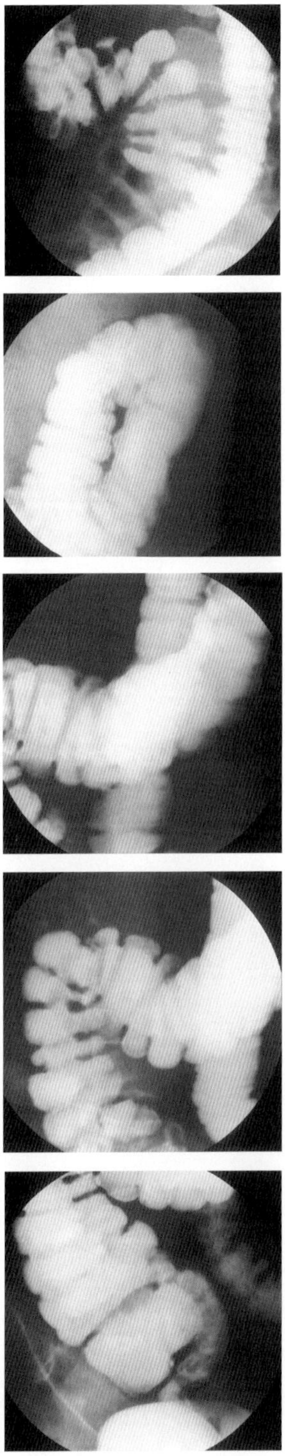

spot film

3 ***Image Remainder of Colon*** *(continued)*

Although the entire colon should be opacified and adequately imaged, spot films of each colonic segment are not routinely obtained with the meticulous detail required for adult examinations (except in precolostomy takedown exams). Because of the nature of the conditions being assessed and the lack of bowel preparation, these images generally do not provide sufficient additional information to justify the increased radiation exposure in the pediatric population. Conditions which would require evaluation of a prepared bowel can be imaged with double contrast technique but are now generally examined endoscopically.

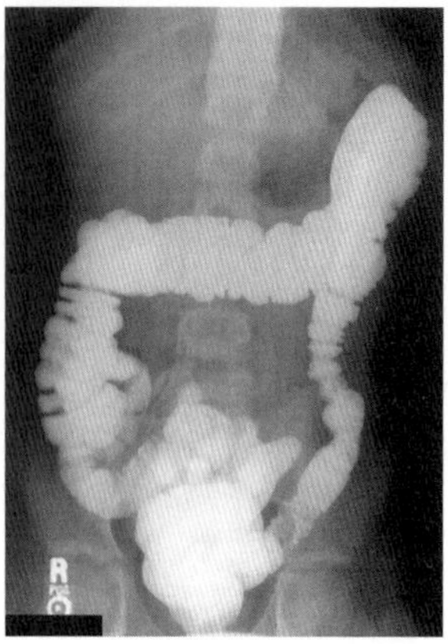

10 × 12
or
30 × 35 cm

4 *Obtain Overhead Film*

Have the technologist obtain an overhead film of the abdomen and pelvis.

TABLETOP
Horizontal

80 kVp

PATIENT
AP

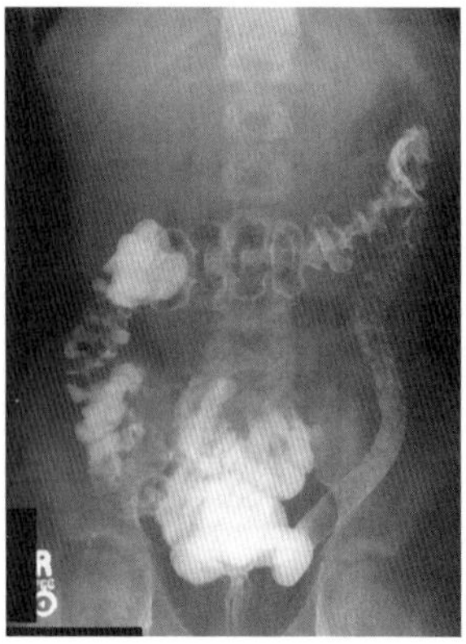

10 × 12
or
30 × 35 cm

5 *Obtain Postevacuation/Drainage Film*

Lower the enema bag below the tabletop height and drain the barium from the colon. Allow the patient to evacuate if possible. Have the technologist obtain an overhead postdrainage/evacuation film of the abdomen. ■

TABLETOP
Horizontal

80 kVp

PATIENT
AP

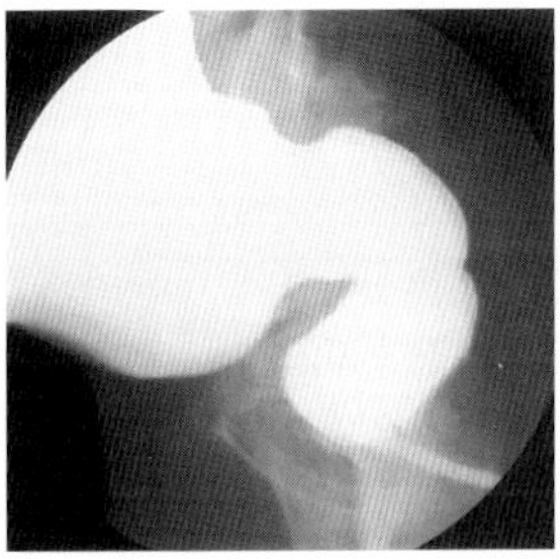

✪ *Single Contrast Enema for Hirschsprung Disease*

Single contrast technique can be utilized in patients with suspected Hirschsprung disease to identify a transition zone.

A lubricated small, straight catheter is carefully inserted in the rectum and secured as described above.

If present, a transition zone is best visualized on lateral images of the rectum during early filling with contrast. Once a transition zone is identified, the examination is generally terminated. Have the technologist obtain AP and lateral overhead films of the filled rectum. The transition zone is often located in the rectum, but can be located anywhere proximally.

If no transition zone is identified, continue filling the colon with contrast and acquire representative spot images with the patient in the supine position. Terminate filling once the cecum is reached. Document the cecal location. Drain the barium from the colon and allow the patient to evacuate if possible.
Have the technologist obtain an overhead post-evacuation/drainage film of the abdomen. ■

TABLETOP
Horizontal

80 kVp

PATIENT
Lat

Air Enema for Intussusception Diagnosis and Reduction

Air reduction of intussusception is an inherently dangerous procedure that should be performed only by radiologists who have been trained specifically in this technique.

INDICATIONS

- Suspected intussusception

CONTRAINDICATIONS

- Pneumoperitoneum
- Delayed diagnosis (over 24 hours) is a relative contraindication to air reduction based on the probability of infarcted bowel
- Radiologist inexperience with air reduction (inexperienced radiologists who must perform intussusception reduction should use the safer contrast enema technique; see specific instructions below)

PATIENT PREPARATION

- Consultation with a pediatric surgeon (who will often be in attendance during the procedure) before attempted reduction
- Intravenous access
- ±Nasogastric tube (patients often vomit after reduction)

SUPPLIES

- Written consent form
- 16–18 Fr Foley catheter with 30 cc balloon or Shiel catheter
- 20 cc syringe (to inflate balloon)
- Insufflator with gauge (preferably with pop-off valve)
- Connector to attach insufflator tubing to Foley catheter
- Lubricating jelly
- Thin and wide tape
- 18 gauge needle (for emergency decompression of tension pneumoperitoneum)

SCOUT FILM

- AP and left lateral decubitus abdomen

SAMPLE DICTATION

Informed and written consent was obtained from the patient's parents. The risks of bowel perforation and possible resulting emergency surgery were discussed. Following consultation with pediatric surgery, an air enema was performed for diagnosis and possible reduction of intussusception. The colon was slowly inflated with air, and an intussusception mass was visualized in the ascending colon. Additional air was carefully administered, and the intussusception was observed to reduce. Reflux of air into multiple loops of small bowel was documented. ■

RADIATION

- Pulsed fluoro: 325 mrad/min
- Spot films: 50 mrad per spot film
  Digital spot films are preferred over cassettes to reduce radiation exposure.

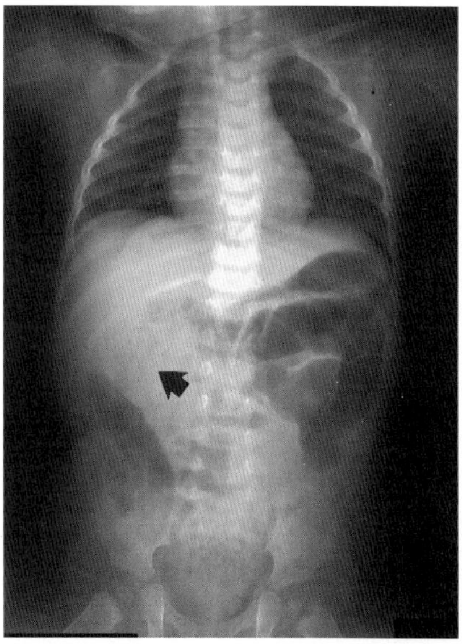

FIGURE 1. *Classical bowel gas pattern seen in patients with intussusception (arrow).*

EXAM

1 *Obtain Informed Consent*

Obtain informed consent from the patient's parents:

1. Risks: bowel perforation, failure of reduction
2. Benefits
3. Alternatives

2 *Prepare Equipment*

Inflate the Foley catheter balloon to assess for integrity and test the manometer. Have an 18 gauge needle immediately available for emergency decompression if a tension pneumoperitoneum develops. Decompression is performed by puncturing through the umbilicus.

3 *Insert Catheter Tip in Rectum*

Connect the tip of the Foley catheter to the insufflator tubing. Immobilize the patient between two sandbags. Gently insert the lubricated catheter tip into the rectum. Secure the catheter to the buttocks and tape the buttocks together to form a seal around the catheter tip.

Under fluoroscopic visualization, carefully inflate the Foley catheter balloon in the rectum with up to 20 cc air.

TABLETOP
Horizontal

70 kVp

PATIENT
PA

4 *Inflate Colon*

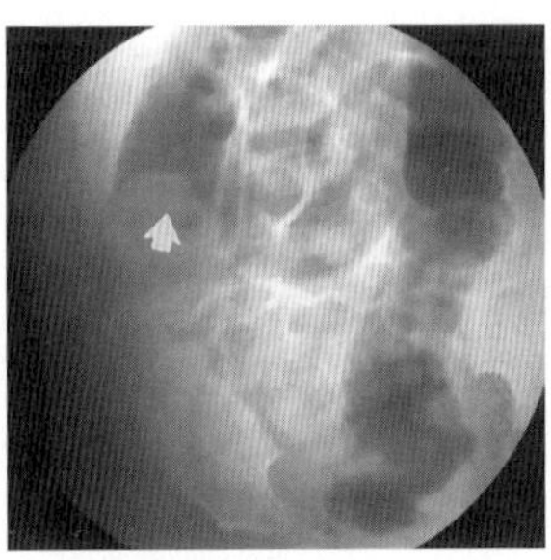

spot film

Place the patient in the supine position. Under fluoroscopic visualization, carefully inflate the colon with air, *maintaining intraluminal pressure of less than 120 mm Hg at all times.* It is necessary to be able to release pressure quickly, as a valsalva maneuver will suddenly increase intraluminal pressure. It is important to reflux air into the distal ileum to avoid missing an intussusception. If an intussusception is encountered, obtain documentation with spot films.

TABLETOP
Horizontal

PATIENT
AP

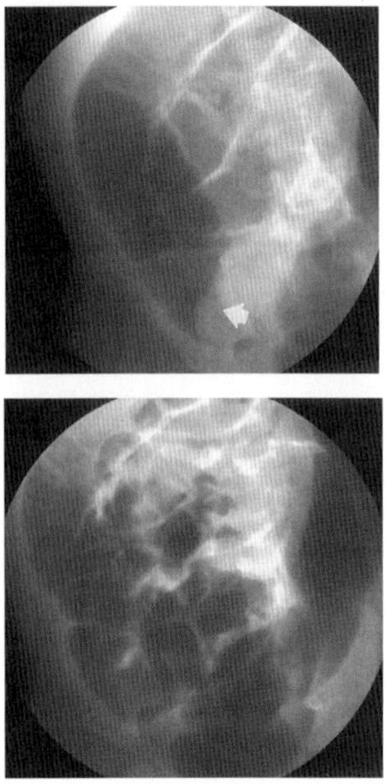

spot film

5 *Reduce Intussusception*

Once an intussusception is diagnosed, reduction can be attempted by continued insufflation of air under fluoroscopic visualization.

The intussusception mass will be observed to move proximally as it is being reduced.

Successful reduction is indicated by retrograde filling of the small bowel with air and disappearance of the intussusception mass.

TABLETOP
Horizontal

PATIENT
AP

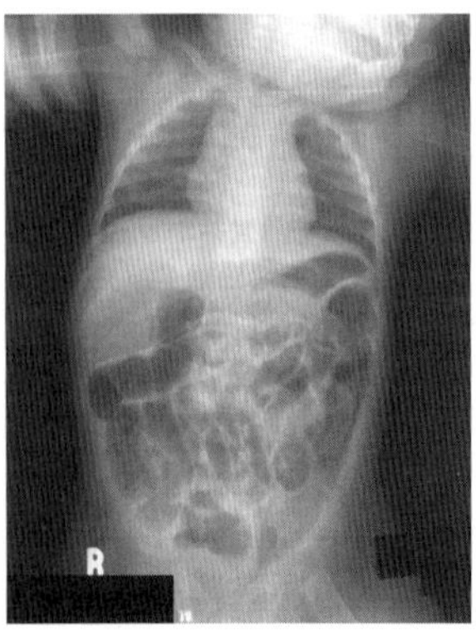

10 × 12
or
30 × 35 cm

6 *Obtain Overhead Film*

Successful reduction of intussusception or absence of intussusception should be documented by demonstrating filling of small bowel loops with air. The postprocedure film should be carefully inspected for evidence of recurrent intussusception or pneumoperitoneum.

The recurrence rate of intussusception is up to 10% and most frequently occurs within 48 hours after reduction. Thus, patients are usually admitted for observation following reduction. ■

TABLETOP
Horizontal

PATIENT
AP

✪ *Contrast Enema for Intussusception Diagnosis and Reduction*

Alternatively, intussusception diagnosis and reduction can be performed with contrast enemas. Both barium and water-soluble contrast agents have been used successfully. The balloon on the enema tip is not inflated. Traditionally, the bag of contrast is suspended no more than 3 feet above the tabletop, and up to three attempted reductions can be performed, with each attempt lasting for up to 3 minutes.

Successful reduction of intussusception or absence of intussusception should be documented by demonstrating reflux of contrast into the terminal ileum. ■

TABLETOP
Horizontal

80 kVp

PATIENT
AP

Pediatric Voiding Cystourethrogram

INDICATIONS

- Febrile urinary tract infection
- Abnormal renal ultrasound
- Follow-up of known vesicoureteral reflux
- Follow-up of pyelonephritis

CONTRAINDICATIONS

- Active infection
- Sufficient sedation to impede normal voiding

PATIENT PREPARATION

- None

SUPPLIES

- 500+ cc 8% iodine uroradiologic contrast (e.g., Cysto-Conray II, Cystografin Dilute)
- 18 gauge needle (to vent contrast bottle)
- Plastic tubing with flow control device
- Luer to catheter tubing adapter
- Sterile gloves (use latex-free gloves for latex allergy/precautions)
- Sterile drape (±fenestration, depending on gender)
- Povidone-iodine solution (e.g., Betadine)
- Sterile cotton balls
- Basin (to collect residual urine)
- 5–8 Fr pediatric feeding tube
- 2% viscous lidocaine gel
- Specimen vial
- Cloth tape
- ±Towel (to collect voided contrast)
- ±Disposable urinal

SCOUT FILM

- KUB/babygram

SAMPLE DICTATION

A 5 Fr pediatric feeding tube was placed through the urethra, and the urinary bladder was filled with 350 cc Cystografin Dilute by gravity. The bladder is normal in size and has normal contours. No filling defects are identified. Voiding images reveal a normal-appearing urethra. There was no vesicoureteral reflux or significant postvoid residual. ■

RADIATION

- Pulsed fluoro: 325 mrad/min
- Spot films: 50 mrad per spot film
  Digital spot films are preferred over cassettes to reduce radiation exposure.

TABLE 1. *Grades of Vesicoureteral Reflux*

GRADE	DESCRIPTION
I	Reflux limited to distal ureter
II	Reflux into collecting system without dilatation or caliceal blunting
III	Reflux into collecting system with mild dilatation or caliceal blunting
IV	Reflux into collecting system with moderate dilatation or caliceal blunting
V	Reflux into collecting system with severe dilatation, caliceal blunting, and tortuous ureters

EXAM

1 *Catheterize Urinary Bladder*

Using sterile technique, catheterize the urinary bladder with a pediatric feeding tube that is lubricated with lidocaine gel. Obtain a clean urine specimen if needed. Drain any residual urine from the bladder so that it does not dilute the contrast. Secure the catheter to the patient's skin using a small amount of tape.

Place an adhesive radiopaque marker on the image intensifier to indicate the patient's right side.

TABLETOP
Horizontal

PATIENT
AP

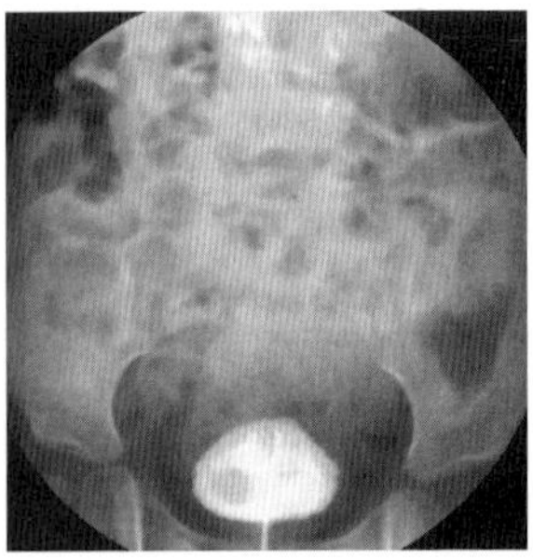

spot film

2 *Instill Contrast*

Connect the contrast-primed tubing to the catheter and begin filling by gravity. Record the amount of contrast administered. The expected bladder volume in patients up to age 13 can be approximated:

$$\text{Expected bladder volume} = (\text{age in years} + 2) \times 30 \text{ cc}$$

Obtain an AP image of the bladder during early filling.

TABLETOP
Horizontal

Pulsed fluoro
7.5 fr/sec
70 kVp

PATIENT
AP

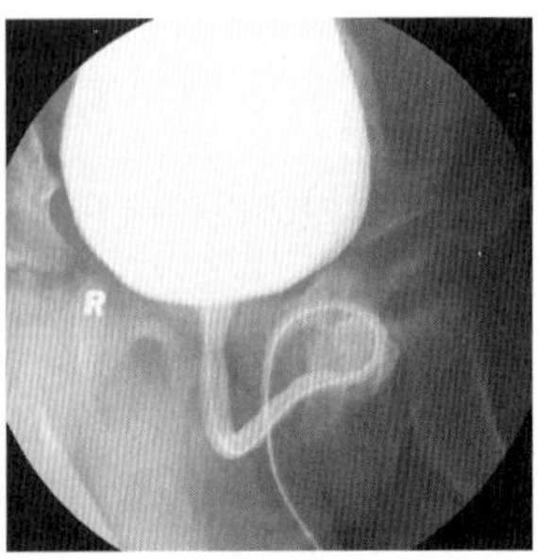

spot film

3 *Perform Cyclic Voiding*

Cyclic voiding should be performed in patients less than 1 year of age to elicit vesicoureteral reflux. The patient will partially void with the catheter in place. The bladder should then be refilled with contrast.

TABLETOP
Horizontal

PATIENT
AP

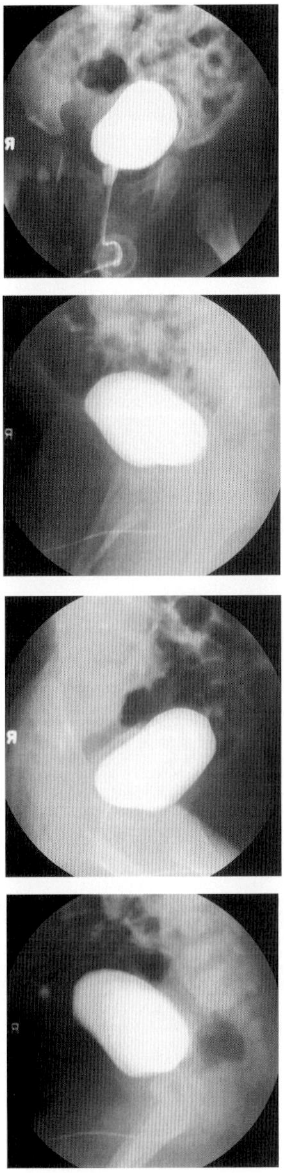

spot film

4 *Image Bladder*

Once the bladder appears maximally filled, stop filling with contrast. This can be assessed by observing that the patient appears uncomfortable or contrast stops flowing spontaneously. Image the bladder in the following positions:

1. AP
2. RPO (focusing on vesicoureteral junction)
3. LPO (focusing on vesicoureteral junction)
4. Lateral

It is important to image the bladder dome to evaluate for urachal abnormalities, as well as the bladder base to evaluate for masses.

TABLETOP

Horizontal

PATIENT

AP

RPO

LPO

Lat

5 *Assess for Vesicoureteral Reflux*

Visualize the bladder and observe for vesicoureteral reflux. Obtain images if reflux is seen, documenting the most superior extent of the reflux.

TABLETOP

Horizontal

PATIENT

AP

±Obliques

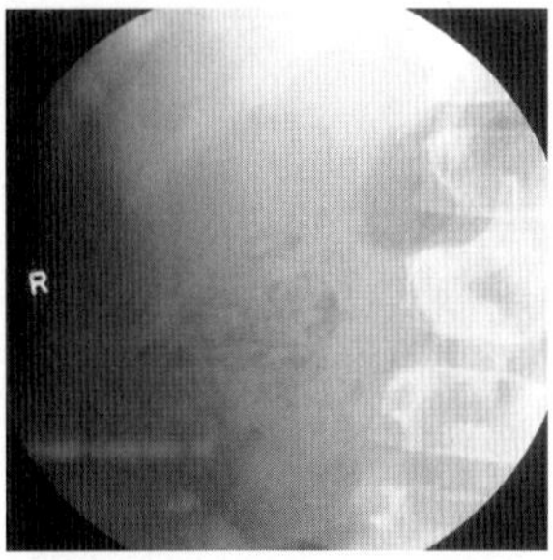

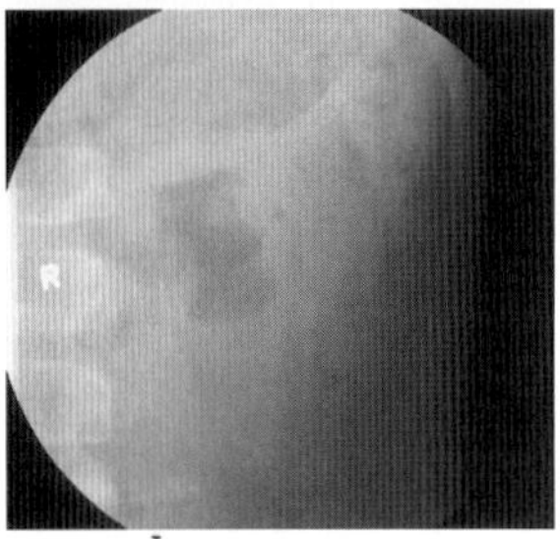

spot film

6 *Image Kidneys*

Image each kidney, looking for the presence of contrast from vesicoureteral reflux.

TABLETOP
Horizontal

PATIENT
AP

7 *Position Patient for Urethrogram*

If the patient is male, turn him RPO or LPO to improve visualization of the urethra.

If the patient is female, place her in the AP position. If vaginal reflux is suspected, this can be confirmed in the lateral position.

Position the fluoroscope so that the base of the bladder can be seen. It is often necessary to use rapid-sequence imaging to obtain images of the opacified urethra.

Place an absorbent towel near the urethra to collect the voided contrast.

Older children can be positioned upright, like adults, and void into a disposable urinal.

TABLETOP
Horizontal
Vertical

PATIENT
♂ RPO/LPO
♀ AP

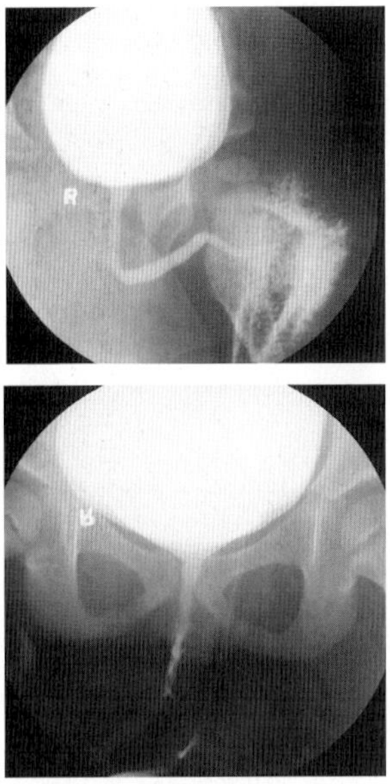

spot film

8 *Image Urethra*

Voiding can be elicited by continued filling of the bladder with contrast or by pouring a small amount of lukewarm water on the perineum.

As the urethra fills with contrast, begin imaging. Image the entire urethra.

TABLETOP

Horizontal

Vertical

Rapid-seq

2 fr/sec

PATIENT

♂ RPO/LPO

♀ AP

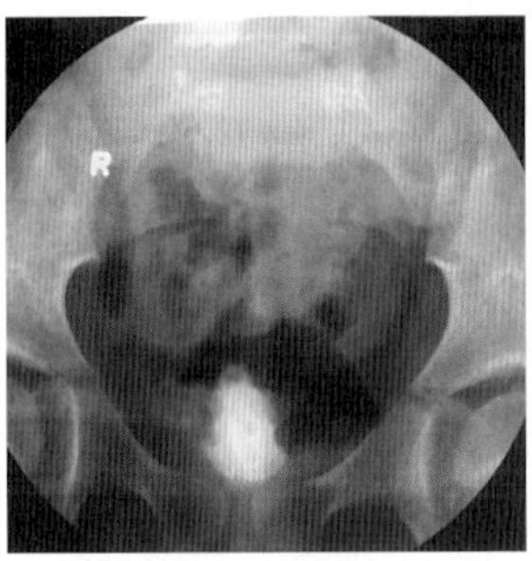

spot film

9 *Image Postvoid Bladder*

Obtain one image of the postvoid bladder. Calculate the postvoid residual (PVR):

$$PVR = (\text{contrast instilled}) - (\text{contrast voided})$$

This image is generally obtained fluoroscopically, but can be obtained by the technologist as an overhead image (at the expense of additional radiation). ■

TABLETOP

Horizontal

Vertical

PATIENT

AP

Pediatric Intravenous Urogram

INDICATIONS

- Suspected aberrant ureteral or renal collecting system anatomy

CONTRAINDICATIONS

- Renal insufficiency (BUN > 30, Cr > 1.5)
- Severe prior contrast reaction

PATIENT PREPARATION

- Premedication if there is a history of prior mild contrast reactions
- A carbonated beverage can be consumed immediately prior to the examination to fill the stomach and allow visualization of the kidneys.
- NPO 2–4 hours (depending on age) prior to exam

SUPPLIES

- ± Written consent form
- Nonionic pediatric excretory urography contrast (e.g., Isovue 250/300, Omnipaque 300, Optiray 320, Ultravist 300, Visipaque 270)
- 60 cc syringe (for contrast)
- 18 gauge needle (for drawing contrast)
- 21–23 gauge butterfly needle and tubing
- Alcohol swab
- Tourniquet
- Tape (to secure IV)
- Small bandage

SCOUT FILM

- Babygram/KUB

SAMPLE DICTATION

The scout film reveals no significant abnormalities. After informed consent was obtained from the patient's parents, 32 cc Omnipaque 300 was administered through an antecubital vein. The immediate nephrogram shows equal opacification of both kidneys, which are normal in size, shape, and position. Excretion of contrast into the collecting systems is normal and equal at 10 minutes. The collecting systems appear normal, without filling defects or displacement. The ureters were fully opacified and are normal in course and caliber. There was no significant postvoid retention of contrast. ■

RADIATION

- Pulsed fluoro: 325 mrad/min
- Spot films: 50 mrad per spot film

EXAM

1 *Obtain Informed Consent*

Ask about previous contrast reactions and obtain written consent if necessary. Explain the possible side effects of intravenous contrast material.

Verify that the patient does not have impaired renal function. Some institutions require serum BUN/creatinine measurements on all patients within 4 weeks.

2 *Inject Contrast*

Calculate the needed quantity of contrast material using the patient's weight and the manufacturer's recommended dosing instructions. As a general rule, the volume of 27–32% iodine nonionic intravascular contrast will roughly equal the patient's weight (in pounds) × 2. More than 50 cc is generally unnecessary.

Flush the IV tubing with contrast. Start an antecubital vein IV and inject the contrast, watching for extravasation.

TABLETOP
Horizontal

PATIENT
AP

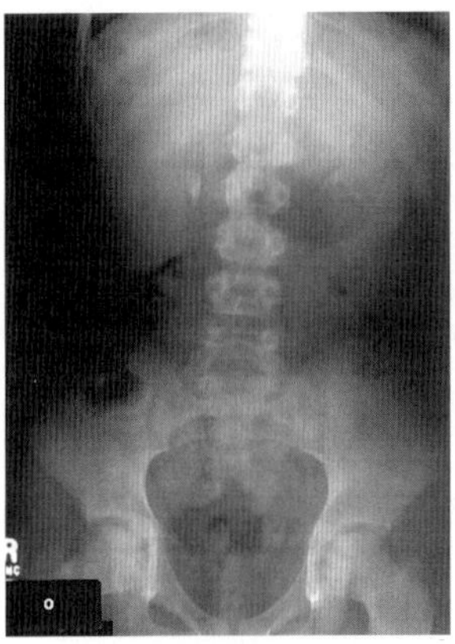

10 × 12
or
14 × 14

3 *Film Immediate Nephrogram*

Have the technologist obtain an overhead immediate nephrogram film.

TABLETOP
Horizontal

65 kVp

PATIENT
AP

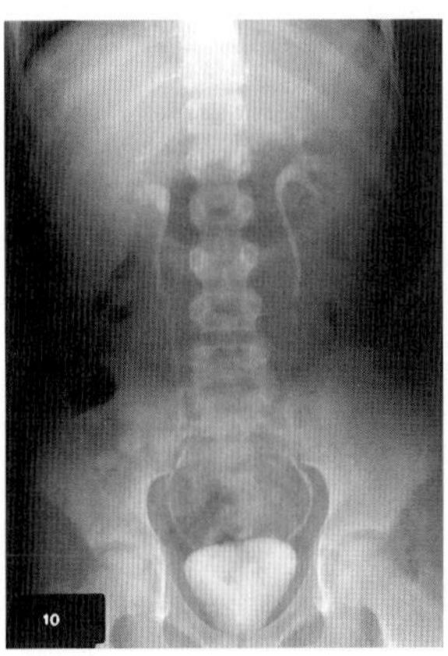

10 × 12
or
14 × 14
or
30 × 35 cm

spot film
mag

4 *Film 10 Minute Image*

Have the technologist obtain a 10 minute overhead film, including the kidneys and ureters.

If the ureters are not sufficiently visualized, they can be imaged fluoroscopically. Contrast that has accumulated in the renal collecting systems can be dumped into the ureters by raising the tabletop to 30–40°. Prone imaging can also help to opacify the ureters.

Obtain spot films to document abnormal ureteral anatomy if necessary. Occasionally, voiding images may be required to define aberrant ureteral anatomy. ■

TABLETOP
Horizontal

65 kVp

PATIENT
AP
±Obliques

PART IX

Miscellaneous Examinations

Jeffrey D. Houston, M.D.
Michael Davis, M.D.

"Sniff" Test (for Diaphragmatic Paralysis)

INDICATIONS

- Suspected diaphragmatic paralysis

CONTRAINDICATIONS

- None

PATIENT PREPARATION

- None

SUPPLIES

- None

SCOUT FILM

- PA/lateral chest x-ray
- Right and left lateral decubitus films if effusions are present

SAMPLE DICTATION

Videofluoroscopic evaluation of diaphragmatic movement was performed. Both hemidiaphragms move in unison, with normal excursion on inspiration and expiration. ■

RADIATION

- Fluoro: 140 mrad/min

EXAM

1 *Prepare Video Recorder*

This exam is primarily a videofluoroscopic procedure. Record the entire exam on videotape.

2 *Observe Diaphragms Independently*

Have the patient inhale and exhale while fluoroscopically observing each hemidiaphragm independently.

A paralyzed diaphragm will have no movement or will have paradoxical movement (movement in the opposite direction). A partially paralyzed diaphragm may have limited movement in the normal direction.

TABLETOP

Horizontal

75 kVp

PATIENT

AP

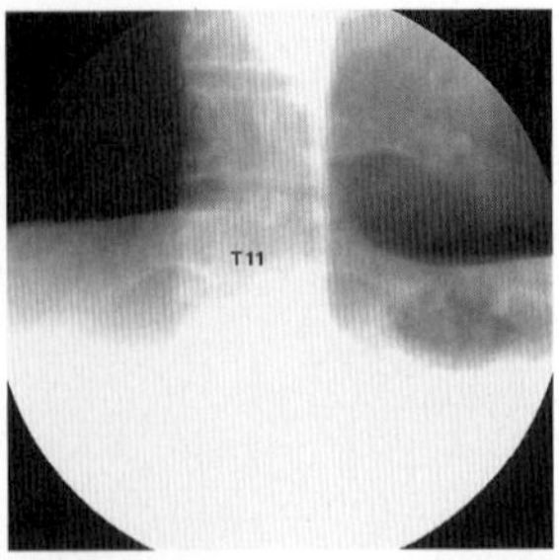

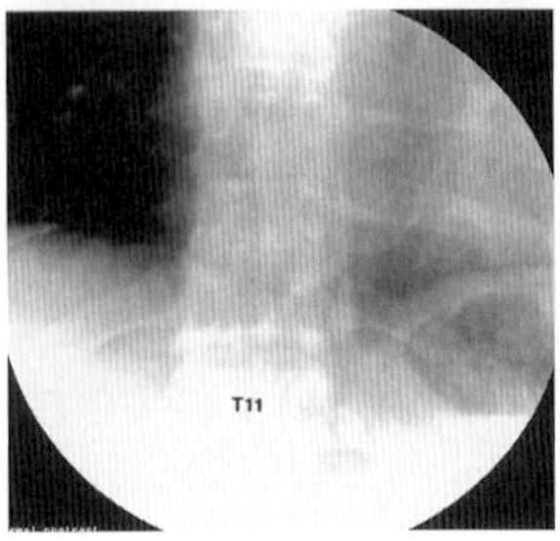

3 *Observe Diaphragms Simultaneously*

Have the patient inhale and exhale while observing both diaphragms simultaneously. If you cannot see both diaphragms at the same time, oblique the patient until you can visualize the medial aspect of each diaphragm.

TABLETOP
Horizontal

PATIENT
AP/RPO

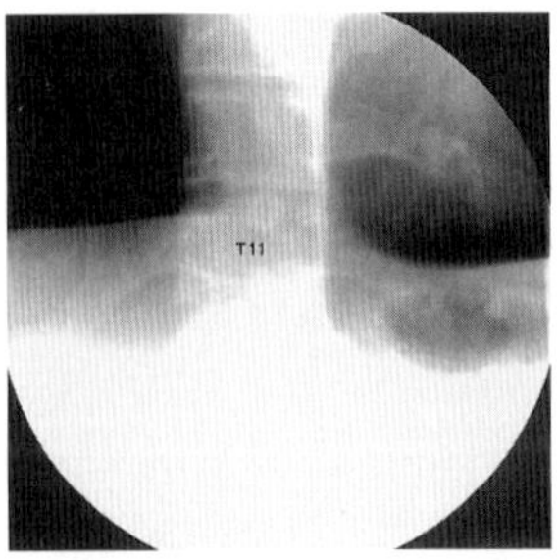

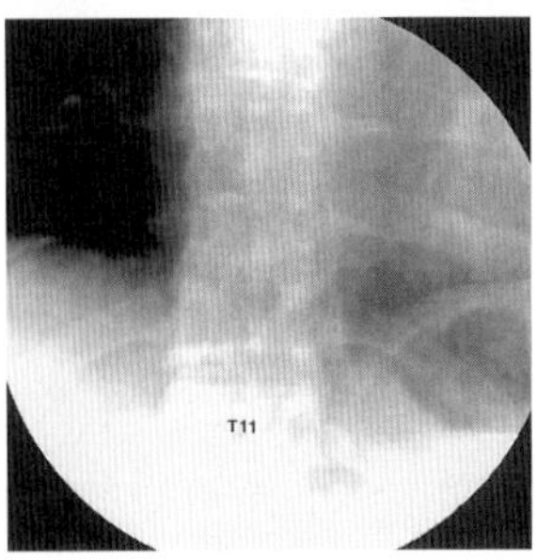

4 *Observe Diaphragms While Sniffing*

Repeat steps 2 and 3 while having the patient inhale rapidly ("sniff") through the nose or pursed lips. ■

TABLETOP
Horizontal

PATIENT
AP/RPO

Cutaneous Fistulogram

INDICATIONS

- Evaluation of cutaneous fistula or sinus tract

CONTRAINDICATIONS

- No common contraindications

PATIENT PREPARATION

- None

SUPPLIES

- 60 cc luer syringe
- 20+ cc 30–40% iodine water-soluble intravascular contrast (e.g., Hypaque-76, MD-76, RenoCal-76)
- 18 gauge needle (for drawing contrast)
- Assortment of Foley catheters
- Luer to tubing adapter

SCOUT FILM

- AP abdomen

SAMPLE DICTATION

An 8 Fr Foley catheter was inserted into the cutaneous fistula opening located in the right lower quadrant. Approximately 20 cc RenoCal-76 was injected into the fistula, revealing a tract that extended into the sigmoid colon. ■

RADIATION

- Fluoro: 100 mrad/min
- Spot films: 10 mrad per spot film

EXAM

1 *Cannulate Cutaneous Opening*

Assess the size of the fistula at the skin surface and select the largest catheter possible for a secure fit. Connect the contrast-filled syringe and flush the tube free of air. Insert the catheter tip into the cutaneous opening as far as it can be inserted without significant resistance.

Secure the syringe and then bring the fluoroscope into position, removing soiled gloves before touching the fluoroscope.

TABLETOP

Horizontal

PATIENT

Various

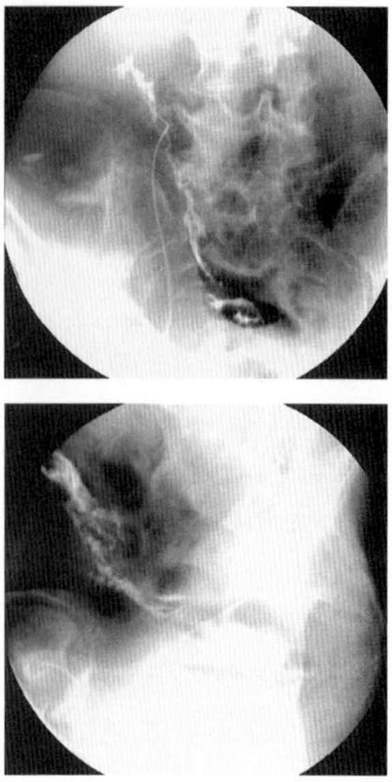

spot film
or
10 × 12
1 on 1

2 *Inject Contrast and Image Tract*

Begin injecting contrast and obtain spot images as the tract fills.

If the colon or small bowel begins to fill, obtain just enough images to document the location.

If the tract does not connect to any organ and ends blindly, obtain AP and lateral views.

If the tract fills an abscess cavity, obtain AP and lateral views. The lateral view will indicate the depth of the abscess.

TABLETOP
Horizontal

75 kVp

PATIENT
Various

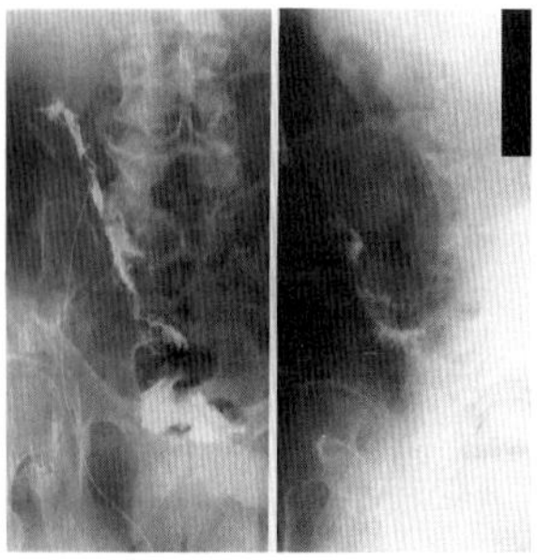

14 × 14
1–2 on 1

3 *Obtain Overhead Films*

Obtain several representative 14 × 14 films or have the technologist obtain an overhead AP 14 × 17 film.

TABLETOP
Horizontal

75 kVp

PATIENT
Various

4 *Remove Catheter*

After reviewing the images, remove the catheter and place a clean dressing on the cutaneous opening. ■

Appendices

Premedication for Contrast Allergy

Management of Contrast Reactions

Iodinated Contrast Media—Intravascular (Ionic)

Iodinated Contrast Media—Intravascular (Nonionic)

Iodinated Contrast Media—Gastrointestinal (Ionic)

Iodinated Contrast Media—Urologic (Ionic)

Barium Sulfate Formulations

Methylcellulose Solutions

Premedication for Contrast Allergy

TABLE 1. *Standard Pretreatment Regimen for Individuals with Prior Intravenous Contrast Reactions (in Hours Prior to Exam)*

HOURS PRIOR TO EXAM	MEDICATIONS
13	Prednisone 50 mg po
7	Prednisone 50 mg po
1	Prednisone 50 mg po Diphenhydramine 50 mg po or IM

TABLE 2. *Emergency Pretreatment Regimen for Individuals with Prior Intravenous Contrast Reactions*

HOURS PRIOR TO EXAM	MEDICATIONS
4 (if possible)	Hydrocortisone 200 mg IV
1	Diphenhydramine 50 mg po or IM

TABLE 3. *Effect of Pretreatment on the Prevalence of Contrast Reactions in Persons Who Previously Had Reactions to Intravenous Contrast*

PRETREATMENT REGIMEN	REACTION PREVALENCE	REFERENCES
None	17–35%	Fischer HW, Doust VL. An evaluation of pretesting in the problem of serious and fatal reactions to excretory urography. *Radiology* 1972; 103:497–501. Witten DM. Reactions to urographic contrast media. *JAMA* 1975; 231:974–977.
Prednisone Diphenhydramine (ionic contrast)	5–11%	Greenberger PA, Patterson R, Tapio CM. Prophylaxis against repeated radiocontrast media reactions in 857 cases. *Arch Intern Med* 1985; 145:2197–2200. Kelly JF, Patterson R, Lieberman P, Mathison DA, Sevenson DD. Radiographic contrast media studies in high-risk patients. *J Allergy Clin Immunol* 1978; 62:181–184.
Prednisone Diphenhydramine (nonionic contrast)	0.5%	Greenberger PA, Patterson R. The prevention of immediate generalized reactions to radiocontrast media in high-risk patients. *J Allergy Clin Immunol* 1991; 87:867–872.

Management of Contrast Reactions

TABLE 1. Treatment Regimens for Acute Contrast Reactions

SIGNS AND SYMPTOMS	TREATMENT	DOSE (ADULT)	DOSE (CHILDREN)	TREATMENT INTERVAL	TREATMENT PRECAUTIONS
Nausea/vomiting					
Transient	Supportive				
Severe	Prochlorperazine (Compazine)	5–10 mg IM/IV	>2 yr: 0.13mg/kg IM	q 3–4 hr	Drowsiness
Urticaria					
Transient	Supportive				
Protracted	Diphenhydramine (Benadryl)	25–50 mg IV/IM	1.25 mg/kg IV/IM	q 2–3 hr	Drowsiness
Profound	Cimetidine (Tagamet) *or*	300 mg IV slow diluted	5–10 mg/kg IV slow diluted	q 6–8 hr	Drowsiness
	Ranitidine (Zantac)	50 mg IV slow diluted	Use not established	q 6–8 hr	
Bronchospasm	Oxygen	3 L/min	3 L/min		
Mild-moderate	1:1000 epinephrine	0.1–0.2 mg sc	0.01–0.02 mg/kg sc (max 0.2 mg)	q 10–15 min	Nonsel. β-blocker
Accelerating	1:10,000 epinephrine	0.1 mg IV slow	0.01 mg/kg IV slow (max 0.1 mg)	q 2–3 min	Nonsel. β-blocker
Wheezing	Albuterol (Proventil) *or* Metaproterenol (Alupent) *or* Terbutaline (Brethaire)	2 inhalations	1–2 inhalations (if possible)	q 4–6 hr	Proper inhalation technique
Hypotension					
nml sinus rhythm/ tachycardia	IV fluids (e.g., normal saline, Ringer's)	1–2 L IV rapid	10–20 mL/kg IV rapid	Per blood pres/urine output	Fluid overload
Bradycardia	IV fluids + atropine	1 mg IV push	0.02 mg/kg IV (max 0.6 mg)	q 3–5 min to 2–3 mg	Monitor pulse
Seizures					
Isolated	See hypotension				
Multiple	Diazepam (Valium)	5–10 mg IV	0.2–0.5 mg/kg IV	q 20 min	Respir. depression

Routes of administration: IV—intravenous, IM—intramuscular, sc—subcutaneous.

Adapted from Bush WH, Swanson DP. Acute reactions to intravascular contrast media: Types, risk factors, recognition, and specific treatment. AJR 1991; 157:1153–1161.

Iodinated Contrast Media—Intravascular (Ionic)

TABLE 1. Intravascular Ionic Iodinated Contrast Media (in Order of Increasing Iodine Concentration)

TRADE NAME	MANUFACTURER	% IODINE CONC.	IODINE (mg/mL)	OSMOLALITY (mOsm/kg)
Reno-DIP Diatrizoate Meglumine 30%	Bracco Diagnostics	14.1	141	566
Conray 30 Iothalamate Meglumine 30%	Mallinckrodt	14.1	141	~600
Conray 43 Iothalamate Meglumine 43%	Mallinckrodt	20.2	202	~1000
Conray Iothalamate Meglumine 60%	Mallinckrodt	28.2	282	1400
Reno-60 Diatrizoate Meglumine 60%	Bracco Diagnostics	28.2	282	1404
Hypaque Meglumine 60% Diatrizoate Meglumine 60%	Nycomed Amersham	28.2	282	1415
Renografin-60 Diatrizoate Meglumine 52% Diatrizoate Sodium 8%	Bracco Diagnostics	29.25	292.5	1450
Hypaque Sodium 50% Diatrizoate Sodium 50%	Nycomed Amersham	30	300	1515
Hexabrix Ioxaglate Meglumine 39.3% Ioxaglate Sodium 19.6%	Mallinckrodt	32	320	~600
MD-76 Diatrizoate Meglumine 66% Diatrizoate Sodium 10%	Mallinckrodt	37	370	1551
RenoCal-76 Diatrizoate Meglumine 66% Diatrizoate Sodium 10%	Bracco Diagnostics	37	370	1870
Hypaque-76 Diatrizoate Meglumine 66% Diatrizoate Sodium 10%	Nycomed Amersham	37	370	2016
Vascoray Diatrizoate Meglumine 52% Diatrizoate Sodium 26%	Mallinckrodt	40	400	~400
Conray 400 Iothalamate Sodium 66.8%	Mallinckrodt	40	400	~2300

Iodinated Contrast Media—Intravascular (Nonionic)

TABLE 1. *Intravascular Nonionic Iodinated Contrast Media (in Order of Increasing Iodine Concentration)*

TRADE NAME	MANUFACTURER	% IODINE CONC.	IODINE (mg/mL)	OSMOLALITY (mOsm/kg)
Omnipaque 140 Iohexol 30%	Nycomed Amersham	14	140	322
Ultravist 150 Iopromide 31%	Berlex Laboratories	15	150	328
Optiray 160 Ioversol 34%	Mallinckrodt	16	160	355
Omnipaque 180 Iohexol 39%	Nycomed Amersham	18	180	408
Isovue-200 Iopamidol 41%	Bracco Diagnostics	20	200	413
Isovue-M 200 Iopamidol 41%	Bracco Diagnostics	20	200	413
Omnipaque 210 Iohexol 45%	Nycomed Amersham	21	210	460
Optiray 240 Ioversol 51%	Mallinckrodt	24	240	502
Omnipaque 240 Iohexol 52%	Nycomed Amersham	24	240	520
Ultravist 240 Iopromide 50%	Berlex Laboratories	24	240	483
Isovue-250 Iopamidol 51%	Bracco Diagnostics	25	250	524
Visipaque 270 Iodixanol 55%	Nycomed Amersham	27	270	290
Oxilan 300 Ioxilan 62%	Cook Imaging	30	300	585
Ultravist 300 Iopromide 62%	Berlex Laboratories	30	300	607
Isovue-300 Iopamidol 61%	Bracco Diagnostics	30	300	616
Isovue-M 300 Iopamidol 61%	Bracco Diagnostics	30	300	616
Optiray 300 Ioversol 64%	Mallinckrodt	30	300	651
Omnipaque 300 Iohexol 65%	Nycomed Amersham	30	300	672
Visipaque 320 Iodixanol 65%	Nycomed Amersham	32	320	290

(continued)

TABLE 1. *Intravascular Nonionic Iodinated Contrast Media (in Order of Increasing Iodine Concentration) (Continued)*

TRADE NAME	MANUFACTURER	% IODINE CONC.	IODINE (mg/mL)	OSMOLALITY (mOsm/kg)
Optiray 320 Ioversol 68%	Mallinckrodt	32	320	702
Oxilan 350 Ioxilan 73%	Cook Imaging	35	350	695
Optiray 350 Ioversol 74%	Mallinckrodt	35	350	792
Omnipaque 350 Iohexol 76%	Nycomed Amersham	35	350	844
Isovue 370 Iopamidol 76%	Bracco Diagnostics	37	370	796
Ultravist 370 Iopromide 77%	Berlex Laboratories	37	370	774

Iodinated Contrast Media—Gastrointestinal (Ionic)

TABLE 1. Gastrointestinal Ionic Iodinated Contrast Media (in Order of Increasing Iodine Concentration)

TRADE NAME	MANUFACTURER	% IODINE CONC.	IODINE (mg/mL)	OSMOLALITY (mOsm/kg)
Gastrografin Diatrizoate Meglumine 66% Diatrizoate Sodium 10%	Bracco Diagnostics	36.7	367	1940
MD-Gastroview Diatrizoate Meglumine 66% Diatrizoate Sodium 10%	Mallinckrodt	36.7	367	2000
Hypaque Sodium Oral Powder Diatrizoate Sodium	Nycomed Amersham	Powder	Powder	Powder

Iodinated Contrast Media—Urologic (Ionic)

TABLE 1. *Urologic Ionic Iodinated Contrast Media (in Order of Increasing Iodine Concentration)*

TRADE NAME	MANUFACTURER	% IODINE CONC.	IODINE (mg/mL)	OSMOLALITY (mOsm/kg)
Cysto-Conray II Iothalamate Meglumine 17.2%	Mallinckrodt	8.1	81	~400
Cystografin Dilute Diatrizoate Meglumine 18%	Bracco Diagnostics	8.5	85	349
Cystografin Diatrizoate Meglumine 30%	Bracco Diagnostics	14	141	556
Cysto-Conray Iothalamate Meglumine 43%	Mallinckrodt	20.2	202	~1000

Barium Sulfate Formulations

TABLE 1. Barium Sulfate Formulations (Listed by Indication and Increasing Weight-Volume)

TRADE NAME	MANUFACTURER	INDICATION	% W/V
Intropaste	Lafayette Pharmaceuticals	Esophageal paste	70% w/v
E-Z Paste	E-Z-EM	Esophageal paste	100% w/v
Liquid Barosperse	Lafayette Pharmaceuticals	Single contrast UGI	60% w/v
Liquid E-Z-Paque	E-Z-EM	Single contrast UGI	60% w/v
Bear-E-Yum GI	Lafayette Pharmaceuticals	Single contrast UGI	60% w/v
Liquid Sol-O-Pake	E-Z-EM	Single contrast UGI	72% w/v
Tonopaque	Lafayette Pharmaceuticals	Single contrast UGI	Powder (17–100% w/v)
Barosperse	Lafayette Pharmaceuticals	Single contrast UGI	Powder (17–110% w/v)
E-Z-Paque	E-Z-EM	Single contrast UGI	Powder (45–65% w/v)
Sol-O-Pake	E-Z-EM	Single contrast UGI	Powder (45–65% w/v)
Ultra-R	E-Z-EM	Single contrast UGI	Powder (45–65% w/v)
EntroEase	Lafayette Pharmaceuticals	See-through SB	13% w/v
Liquid Entero Vu	E-Z-EM	See-through SB	13% w/v
EntroEase Dry	Lafayette Pharmaceuticals	See-through SB	Powder (13% w/v)
Entero Vu	E-Z-EM	See-through SB	Powder (13% w/v)
Entrobar	Lafayette Pharmaceuticals	Single contrast SB	50% w/v
Entero-H	E-Z-EM	Single contrast SB	Powder (80% w/v)
Digital HD	Lafayette Pharmaceuticals	Double contrast UGI	Powder (175% w/v)
Digibar 190	E-Z-EM	Double contrast UGI	Powder (190% w/v)
HD 200 Plus	Lafayette Pharmaceuticals	Double contrast UGI	Powder (225% w/v)
Liqui-Coat HD	Lafayette Pharmaceuticals	Double contrast UGI	210% w/v
Maxibar	E-Z-EM	Double contrast UGI	210% w/v
Enhancer	Lafayette Pharmaceuticals	Double contrast UGI	Powder (225% w/v)
Baricon	Lafayette Pharmaceuticals	Double contrast UGI	Powder (230% w/v)
E-Z-HD	E-Z-EM	Double contrast UGI	Powder (250% w/v)
Pediatric Bear-E-Bag	Lafayette Pharmaceuticals	Single contrast BE	Powder (13–33% w/v)
Solo-O-Pake Enema Bag	E-Z-EM	Single contrast BE	Powder (14–25% w/v)
Barobag Enema Kit	Lafayette Pharmaceuticals	Single contrast BE	Powder (15–44% w/v)
E-Z-Paque Enema Bag	E-Z-EM	Single contrast BE	Powder (14–25% w/v)
HD 85	Lafayette Pharmaceuticals	Double contrast BE	85% w/v
E-Z-AC	E-Z-EM	Double contrast BE	100% w/v
Flo-Coat	Lafayette Pharmaceuticals	Double contrast BE	100% w/v
Imager ac	Lafayette Pharmaceuticals	Double contrast BE	100% w/v
Liquid Polibar	E-Z-EM	Double contrast BE	100% w/v
Medebar Plus	Lafayette Pharmaceuticals	Double contrast BE	100% w/v
Liquid Polibar Plus	E-Z-EM	Double contrast BE	105% w/v
Anatrast	Lafayette Pharmaceuticals	Defecography	100% w/v
Evacu-Paste	E-Z-EM	Defecography	100% w/v

% weight-volume (% w/v) = *grams of $BaSO_4$ + sufficient volume of H_2O to produce 100 mL*
% weight-weight (% w/w) = *grams of $BaSO_4$ + sufficient weight of H_2O to produce 100 g*

TABLE 2. *Barium Sulfate Tablets for Evaluating Esophageal Strictures*

TRADE NAME	MANUFACTURER	WEIGHT	DIMENSION
E-Z-Disk	E-Z-EM	10 grains	½ inch/13 mm
Bar-Test	Glenwood	10 grains	½ inch/13 mm

Methylcellulose Solutions

TABLE 1. *Methylcellulose Solutions for Enteroclysis (Listed by Increasing Weight-Volume)*

TRADE NAME	MANUFACTURER	% W/V
MC Solution	E-Z-EM	1% w/v
Entrocel	Lafayette Pharmaceuticals	1.8% w/v (concentrate)

Index

Note: Page numbers followed by f indicate figures; those followed by t indicate tables.